The Revolutionary Trauma Release Process

The Revolutionary Trauma Release Process

Transcend Your Toughest Times

❀ ❀ ❀ ❀ ❀

DAVID BERCELI, PhD

NAMASTE PUBLISHING
Vancouver, Canada

Copyright © 2008 by David Berceli

First Printing 2008   Fifth Printing 2012
Second Printing 2009   Sixth Printing 2014
Third Printing 2010   Seventh Printing 2015

Library and Archives Canada Cataloguing in Publication

Berceli, David, 1953–
    The revolutionary trauma release process : transcend your toughest times / David Berceli.

    ISBN 978-1-897238-40-0 (pbk.)

    1. Post-traumatic stress disorder—Treatment—Popular works. 2. Psychic trauma—Treatment—Popular works. I. Title.

RC552.P67B47 2008   616.85'2106   C2008-902472-9

Published by NAMASTE PUBLISHING, Inc.
PO Box 62084
Vancouver, BC, Canada V6J 4A3
www.namastepublishing.com

```
      ®              MIX
                  Paper from
                  responsible sources
  FSC
  www.fsc.org     FSC® C016245
```

Distributed in North America by PGW, Berkeley, CA
Cover design by Gabreyhl Zintoll
Interior book design and typesetting by Val Speidel

Pages 15–17, Excerpts from "Hell and Back" by Chris Rose 10/22/06 © 2008 The Times-Picayune Publishing Co. All rights reserved. Used with permission of The Times-Picayune.

Printed and bound by Friesens Printing in Canada.

DISCLAIMER: The information presented in this book is selective rather than exhaustive. Medical and psychological information is constantly evolving, and the reader should exercise particular care in forming conclusions based solely on this book.

For these reasons, neither David Berceli nor the publisher assume responsibility or liability arising from any error or omission, or from the use of any information, in this book. In no event shall TRAPS, Trauma Release Process LLC, David Berceli, or Namaste Publishing, Inc. be liable for any direct, indirect, punitive, incidental, special, or consequential damages arising out of or in any way connected with the use of these exercises.

The exercises presented in this book are not intended to cure or heal illnesses associated with trauma, only to release the effects of trauma in the musculature, and they should not be taken to be a substitute for appropriate trauma recovery procedures of a medical or psychological nature. For specific diagnosis, treatment, or courses of action for trauma recovery, the reader should always consult a licensed mental health professional who can discuss personal symptoms and appropriate treatment.

These exercises should not be used by pregnant women, infants, or children. They should also not be used by any individual who has serious medical conditions such as a heart condition, irregular blood pressure, or any other medical condition that requires strict regulation, without the approval and supervision of a medical doctor trained to provide such guidance.

Although this book outlines a self-administered trauma recovery process, specific individuals with fragile psychological defenses, a complex history of repeated or multiple traumas, or those with restricting physical limitations or injuries such as knee, back, pelvic, or other muscle, tendon, or bone injuries should consult their medical professional prior to performing these exercises.

Dedicated to the many people who have blessed me with the opportunity to accompany them in their trauma recovery process.

Contents

Acknowledgments

To HAVE WORKED in so many countries, with such large traumatized populations, has been overwhelming in both challenging and encouraging ways. Without these global human experiences, I could not have learned as much as I have about the collective struggle of humanity.

I have received a great deal of support from friends and family, which has truly sustained me. Among them are my mother and father, sisters Denise and Debi, brothers Frank and Michael, and my sister-in-law Kathy. My dear friends Richard, Michael and Kerry, Riccardo, Bob and Jim, Sherry, Anne, and Robert have always supported me with their loving care and patience. Again and again they have shown me the warmth and encouragement of true and valued friendship, which is an important part of our human potential. These relationships helped sustain me and encourage me to continue my journey of human exploration.

Special thanks go to Constance Kellough, President and Publisher at Namaste Publishing, for seeing the value of this work and opening the door to take it into every corner of the world. Thanks must also be given to my editor David Ord, Namaste Publishing's Editorial Director, who tirelessly guided me through the process of writing in a coherent and meaningful manner.

Foreword

DAVID BERCELI spent much of his career in war zones, including Lebanon, the Palestinian West Bank, Israel, Uganda, Sudan, Yemen, and Ethiopia.

It was in Lebanon that he made a trenchant observation about himself and his co-workers when huddled against the wall in a building being shelled by mortars. He noted that, in response to the concussion of an exploding mortar shell, each person in the room startled and assumed a posture in which their shoulders and hips contracted toward each other as if they were going into a ball. He intuitively recognized this as a universal response to danger and therefore instinctual in all of us.

With his expertise as a therapeutic body worker, David realized that repetitive activation of the muscles that create this flexion could result in tension building up in these muscles. He also surmised that releasing this tension could have many beneficial effects. With careful analysis, David determined that one specific muscle, the psoas, played a large role in this process.

The result is the groundbreaking Trauma Release Process (TRP™) described in this remarkable book. Application of these exercises throughout the world has allowed clients to achieve a sense of release, relaxation, and calmness. Often, even emotional states from old trauma are mitigated.

I met David several years ago through an organization devoted to fostering resiliency and health in returning Iraq veterans. When David told me about his work, I immediately recognized the rationale for the effectiveness of his exercises in healing trauma and chronic back pain through discharging the tension in muscles. Since then we have corresponded and collaborated on many projects devoted to the healing of trauma. I personally have used and taught the Trauma Release Process™ to friends and patients with consistently remarkable results.

The Revolutionary Trauma Release Process is the result of David's long journey of discovering and perfecting this novel and widely applicable form of trauma therapy. It serves as a useful manual for learning these exercises on one's own. One of the unique features of the exercises is that they can be learned and practiced as a therapeutic self-help skill, as well used as an adjunct to other forms of trauma therapy.

Helplessness is a universal state in the trauma victim, and gaining control of their symptoms, their body, and their life is an essential part of the healing process. This book shows how to achieve this.

— Robert Scaer, MD, Author of *The Body Bears the Burden: Trauma, Dissociation, and Disease,* and *The Trauma Spectrum: Hidden Wounds and Human Resiliency.*

PART I

Making Sense of Stress, Anxiety, and Trauma

I

Life Is Traumatic

❁ ❁ ❁ ❁ ❁

A MOTHER WRINGS HER HANDS and breathes erratically. Her ten-year-old son is way late coming home from school.

In another household, a husband arrives home unusually early for supper. He goes to his favorite chair and slumps into it in despair. He has just lost his job.

Elsewhere, a seventeen-year-old throws herself in her mother's lap, confessing between sobs that she can't live without her boyfriend, who has just announced his family is moving to another state.

Throughout our lives, we continually face the possibility of painful experiences. Though some of us lead easier, less stressful lives than others, none of us escape difficult times entirely.

Our tendency is to resist these experiences when they come to us. We don't like difficult experiences, and we certainly don't welcome pain!

We naturally try to run from these challenges. Or, if they already have us in their grip, we fight them.

By resisting what we don't like, we actually compound our discomfort. By being at war with ourselves, we make ourselves anxious and our days stressful. Life gets *more* difficult, and we become even *more* tense.

If we find ourselves in too many difficult situations, we may begin to believe our life is going wrong—that we have somehow messed up. As stress and anxiety increasingly dominate our days, we pay a price. Our wellbeing is compromised. We suffer emotional and mental distress, which can escalate into anguish. Before long, this takes a toll—our energy plummets, and our physical health deteriorates.

However, it's *not the events* that cause the damage to our health. It's *how we respond* to them.

A REALLY DIFFERENT APPROACH

Mahatma Gandhi, Martin Luther King Jr., Mother Teresa, and Nelson Mandela are examples of individuals who survived incredible stress. Each of them suffered a great deal in their lives. Yet, they came through these anxiety-provoking, stressful times in such a way as to change the lives of millions of people.

I had often wondered what made such individuals different from most of us. Were they somehow unique, accessing a level of human potential that only a few on the planet are ever able to access?

As I thought about their lives, I realized that the way they dealt with their truly tough times was different from the way many of us handle such times. These people actually plunged into their most trying experiences, exploring the depths of what had befallen them, feeling the pain of their situation in its immensity, and *staying with* the difficult time they were going through instead of running from it.

Mahatma Gandhi experienced imprisonment and severe hardship, while at the same time being completely misunderstood even by people who loved him. But by staying fully present in what he was experiencing, exploring the pain it brought him and going deeply into it with a great deal of soul searching, he came to realize that "non-violence" was the only answer to the crisis his nation was facing. The result was that India became a free country. How did this profound insight come out of such intense suffering? How did imprisonment produce a message that invited humans to rise to a new level of consciousness?

Martin Luther King Jr. also experienced a great deal of personal and social suffering. His followers wanted to riot and overthrow the government because it tolerated prejudice and discrimination. Like Gandhi, he too explored the painful experiences that presented themselves to him. He went *into* his suffering, searching his soul, and emerged with a realization that "civil disobedience" was the way forward. How did these two simple yet powerful words—words that were to change the consciousness of a nation—arise from such suffering?

When Mother Teresa witnessed the depths of human degradation as she walked the streets of Calcutta, she made a choice to live among the poorest of the poor. Why would she embrace such a difficult lifestyle? Of what benefit was this to her? What did she expect to receive from such sacrifice? As Mother Teresa immersed herself in the suffering surrounding her, she began to see humanity differently. Her life and her words challenged humanity to embrace a higher consciousness. As a result, she was awarded the Nobel Peace Prize, the highest honor that can be conferred upon a human being.

And then there is Nelson Mandela, a man who was imprisoned twenty-seven years for speaking out against apartheid. He simply had wanted to be seen as a human being. After all those years in prison, he could have come out bitter, angry, and even more in conflict with the government of his nation than when he was first incarcerated. After all, the greatest part of his life had been taken away from him against his will. Yet when he was released, he proclaimed a message of "reconciliation." He wanted to bring the abused and the abuser together. It was by learning to see through the eyes of an incredibly difficult experience that such a vision was born, enabling the suffering so many of the people of South Africa had endured to have redeeming benefit for humanity.

Each of these great people of our time, whose lives we will revisit in a later chapter, challenged us to become more ethical, more moral, more loving, and ultimately more human. They demonstrated that by going into our toughest times, and emerging transformed on the other side, we receive an amazing gift of new vision.

In the end, the only difference I could detect between these outstanding individuals and the majority of us is that most of us often tend to run from difficult times, push them away, or pretend they aren't happening. We want to avoid pain and suffering at all cost. But I have become convinced that, in our avoidance, denial, and fear, we push away the very experiences that seek to stimulate the evolution of our consciousness. In fact, we deny ourselves the opportunity to become the person we yearn to be and are ultimately destined to become.

ALIGN YOURSELF WITH WHAT IS

When we do battle with what's happening in our lives, we inflict suffering on ourselves and on those around us. We damage ourselves and we damage our relationships.

This book proposes that resistance to *any* aspect of our lives is counterproductive. Fighting what's happening to us leads only to increased suffering. Realizing this fact invites a different approach.

How can we cope with stressful times in a way that doesn't leave us reeling, doesn't turn life into a battlefield, and doesn't damage our health?

Since we cannot prevent such times, the wise response is simply to *allow* them to be as they are.

Because humans are a living organism on this planet, like other species we are designed to *experience, endure, and survive* stressful episodes. Not only can we survive these experiences, we can also learn from them and adapt. In fact, if humans didn't possess the ability to learn from stressful experiences and adapt, our species would have become extinct. The fact we are still here suggests we have learned from the stress endured by our ancestors and adapted well.

The reality is, there will never be a time when our life is free of situations that trigger stress and provoke anxiety. Once we accept this, we experience a shift within ourselves. We then realize that nothing is going wrong during these times. In fact, we can learn how to use our experiences for our benefit.

WHEN LIFE TURNS UP THE HEAT

Stress and anxiety are not the same, although they are close companions and often trigger each other.

Stress comes from the feeling that a certain set of circumstances *should not be happening*.

When we believe something in our life shouldn't be the way it is, we go into a mindset of resistance. We mentally oppose what's happening. This is the feeling we identify as *stress*. Something has come up, and we want to get it over with, get past it, get it out of the way. In other words, *we are in flight from the way our life is right now*.

Anxiety stems from the feeling that something *should* be happening that clearly isn't.

When we believe something ought to be happening, we yearn for it, ache for it, often to the point that our longing eclipses our ability to enjoy what's presently happening in our lives. Longing for something that isn't happening causes us to be dissatisfied with our life as it is right now. The effect upon our mental wellbeing and our health is the same as that of stress.

In both stress and anxiety, our inner experience is that we want to be somewhere other than where we are. We're not happy, not fulfilled with our life as it is at this moment. So, though we are forced to endure the situation because we can't find a way out, we wish we could flee from it. We are here, but our mind is elsewhere, which constitutes a splitting of our whole self.

Usually we get over such times. When something we perceive to be good happens, we forget what it is that "shouldn't be happening" or "ought to be happening."

The problem with merely "getting past" a stressful or anxious time is that, although life appears to move on, nothing has actually changed. We may have left a particularly difficult situation behind, but *we* remain *the same*. In fact, we have simply reinforced our weakness in the face of stress or anxiety, leaving us even more vulnerable to the next source of distress that comes along. Because it was too overwhelming and we didn't have the skills, we couldn't allow the stressful event to have the transformative effect it could have, and consequently we are as vulnerable as ever to subsequent difficult times. Just how such times can become a gift, transforming us, is the subject of a later chapter.

Initially we may not be able to do anything but run away from life's stress and anxiety because it is too difficult to face. But in due course the universe will invite us to continue exploring our stress until we can deal with it. It seems to have a way of turning up the heat that's just right for us. A new situation comes along, this time predictably of greater severity. As stress and anxiety occur with increasing severity, we eventually find ourselves in great distress. Because the situation stresses our nervous system beyond its usual coping ability, we experience a more serious response whose effects don't leave us so easily.

TRAUMA IS INDIVIDUAL IN NATURE

In addition to stress and anxiety, many of us experience *trauma*. It's not always easy to spot when an individual is in trauma. This is because an episode that may overwhelm one person may not be experienced as overwhelming by another.

Whether an experience proves to be traumatic for a particular individual depends on such factors as the person's age—think of how much more vulnerable a small child is, or an elderly person—the severity of the threat, the degree of physical harm that may be inflicted, the possibility of escape, how accustomed to coping with difficulties the individual is, and the cumulative effect of previous trauma.

For instance, due to the individual's life history, one soldier could experience a battle as traumatizing, while another might experience it as only mildly disturbing. One person in a car accident may be frightened of driving for years afterwards, while another person in the same car recovers from this fear in a few weeks.

Feeling traumatized should never be judged as a weakness in an individual. This is because our reaction to potentially traumatizing situations is instinctual and therefore not under our conscious control. We don't make a conscious decision to feel traumatized—it's an *automatic* response.

In fact, we shall see that *a traumatic reaction is a positive response, not negative*. It's not a display of weakness, but rather the body's attempt to protect itself. The basic emergency alert system of the human organism is activated during these times to promote survival.

Trauma can be experienced physically, mentally, and emotionally. Whether it affects our body, our mind, or our emotions—or all of these simultaneously—it's part and parcel of the human experience. It's impossible to go through life without experiencing some degree of trauma.

Though trauma is an unavoidable aspect of life—the result of the body's courageous defense of itself—it's nonetheless an intense experience and something we would rather avoid because it sends us into shock. Yet, it's an integral aspect of our human experience and our evolutionary journey. No matter how much we try to protect ourselves from traumatic experiences, we can't prevent them from happening.

A SHOCK TO THE SYSTEM

Since it's not widely recognized that trauma serves a purpose in our lives, it's essential that we change the way we view traumatic experiences.

Trauma is common to the human species. Consider the fact that life begins traumatically. We come into the world through the painful process of birth—an experience in which we are squeezed out of shape, pushed, and sometimes even pulled with hard, metallic instruments. It's not a pleasant welcoming at all.

Bursting into the light for the first time in our existence, our entry into the world is a shock to the human organism. A room filled with cold air, bright lights, and the noise of other human beings is a drastic change from the dark, soothing warmth we have become accustomed to in the womb. Making our debut in such a hostile atmosphere, it's no wonder we begin life by bellowing our lungs out.

As infants lying in our crib, we are assaulted by hunger pains, colic, skin rashes, and a host of discomforts we don't understand and don't know how to respond to other than by crying helplessly and vociferously.

In due course we discover the ability to move about. For a time we are unstable in our movements, which means inevitable collisions and crashes into unyielding objects. The shock of toppling over time after time as we attempt to walk is in itself stressful.

As we struggle to find our feet, we are guaranteed that life will be punctuated with bumps on the head, cuts, and grazes—all of which are accompanied by tears, either from the physical pain we incur or from a bruised ego.

LEARNING TO "SUCK IT UP"

The journey toward independence isn't only physically traumatic, it's also emotionally traumatic. In fact, our culture presents us with considerable psycho-emotional trauma—the kind of trauma caused primarily hy social conditioning. Situations that threaten our social self such as rejection, shame, fear of failure, and negative judgment by others cause us to react in the same manner as if we were being threatened physically. The body takes up a position of submission and withdrawal, slumping forward with the head down—the precise posture it assumes when threatened by physical trauma.

When we are very young, trauma often accompanies even the most enjoyable of experiences. For instance, once we begin to play among other children, there's always someone who wants the toy we are playing with. Pretty soon our fun turns to tears, tantrums, and trauma as we are dragged away from the sandpit or our friend's yard by a caregiver, then threatened, yelled at, and perhaps even physically assaulted with a spanking.

Then there is the emotional trauma of entering daycare or kindergarten. Until now secure with a parent or caregiver at home, we are suddenly left for the day among strangers—an experience that finds many of us distraught and wailing, "Mommy, Daddy, don't leave me!"

When we begin school, we are likely to encounter bullying, which has emerged as a scourge of the school playing field—and of the school bus. Few of us make it through our educational years without being bullied. Repeated bullying can be extremely traumatizing for a child.

A case in point. When an African American girl turned eleven, her parents decided to send her across town to a junior high school in a culturally different neighborhood. Her experience up to that point had mostly involved middle class African American and Japanese American families. So when she was put on a bus to attend a school in an all-white, affluent neighborhood, she wasn't prepared for the culture clash she was about to experience.

Her first traumatic experience came when, because her stop was one of the last stops of an already overcrowded school bus, no one wanted her to sit next to them. Since she was perceived as "shy and nerdy," they didn't care to scoot over and allow her to share their seat. Each day, the bus driver ordered one of the students to move over, and even then the young girl found herself with only three inches of seat.

Every day, for fifteen miles, she balanced herself on the edge of the seat so she wouldn't fall into the aisle. Next to her sat a resentful student who had yielded almost no space, but who enjoyed taking advantage of the African American student because she was meek, mild, and non-confrontational.

Unfortunately, kids can be cruel to each other at certain times in their lives. For the one who is being shunned, it's a stressful, anxiety-ridden, traumatic experience. Most days, this young girl cried silently all the way to school.

At school, the culture clash didn't turn out to be as bad as the girl had imagined. She found she had much in common with one of the local girls, and they became friends. But this exposed the local girl to her own traumatic experiences. The kids in her own neighborhood began whispering and laughing as she walked by. Soon they were taunting her, telling her she was a traitor, calling her hateful names that stabbed her heart.

Being a teenager is all about trying to fit in and finding your niche. But when your niche is outside of the box, ostracism is the price—as countless school children experience each and every day.

It's stressful growing up in our schools. Many of our kids exist in a state of high anxiety. All they can do is "suck it up."

Quite apart from threats by other people, just growing up has its growing pains. For instance, we may love to play a sport. But even when we are having fun, our excitement is frequently curtailed by the consequences of the rough and tumble, from which painful bruises, twisted ankles, and even broken bones result.

The teen years are also marked by our entry into puberty with its stressful rites of passage—painful periods, pimples that embarrass, and the inevitable broken heart.

So far we've talked about normal children leading ordinary everyday lives. But another, more sinister face of being a child is found in the maltreatment many youngsters experience—a topic we will investigate in a chapter devoted to post-traumatic stress disorder.

STRESS AND FAMILY LIFE

As adults, we face new stresses and different sources of anxiety. On the job, we run up against a boss who makes our life difficult. A coworker betrays us. Or the company out-sources, then downsizes, and we are let go.

At home we may start a family. Now we experience the trauma of growing up from a different vantage—through our children. As parents, we want to protect our children from pain, but we find we can't.

Juggling career and family—a reality for so many today—can be especially anxiety-provoking. As one mother recalls, "Once my first child was born, all of my beliefs and expectations of what I wanted to achieve in this life evaporated. In my heart and mind, ever since I was a little girl, I had carried a dream of being the first woman CEO of a major corporation, and suddenly my dream was gone. I didn't care about anything but my baby. I wanted to nurse him, read to him, hold him, kiss him— all day long."

Our deepest desires often clash with harsh reality, as this mother discovered. The world of commerce presents many challenges. In the work environment, not only are we deprived of being with our children, we often find ourselves dealing with individuals who play mental games with us. People can make the workplace a place of misery—and do so each day for millions.

The National Institute for Occupational Safety and Health reports that 40% of workers find their job to be stressful, and in many cases extremely stressful. A full quarter of the labor force identify their job as the primary source of stress in their life. Almost as many have shed tears over workplace stress. Some 19% have quit a job and 29% have yelled at fellow workers because of stress. In fact, 42% admit that yelling and verbal abuse are commonplace in their work environment. It's no wonder the *Journal of Occupational and Environmental Medicine* reports that health care expenditures are almost 50% greater for workers who experience high levels of stress.

Though no one is immune to trauma, once we recognize that a traumatic experience can serve a valuable purpose in our lives—and that we do not have to live in perpetual trauma after its work is done—we no longer create for ourselves the added suffering that comes from resistance to trauma.

By accepting trauma as an inevitable part of being human, we allow it to have its transformative effect on us.

2

Insight from
Hurricane Katrina

❀ ❀ ❀ ❀ ❀

A COMMON RESPONSE TO TRAUMA is depression. If the trauma is severe enough, an individual may find themselves in a living hell with seemingly no way of escape.

A case in point is New Orleans *Times-Picayune* columnist Chris Rose, who used to believe depression and anxiety were "pretty much a load of hooey." In fact, Rose writes, "I never accorded any credibility to the idea that such conditions were medical in nature."

Rose no longer feels this way. "Not since I fell down the rabbit hole myself," he confessed in the wake of journeying "to the edge of the post-Katrina abyss."

Says Rose, "I had crying jags and fetal positionings and other 'episodes.' One day last fall, while the city was still mostly abandoned, I passed out on the job, fell face first into a tree, snapped my glasses in half, gouged a hole in my forehead and lay unconscious on the side of the road for an entire afternoon."

Another time, Rose had a meltdown at a gas station. He found he simply couldn't get out of his car to fill the gas tank because of the presence of other people at the pumps.

This meltdown came on the heels of his increasing withdrawal from social interaction. He had stopped going to the grocery store weeks earlier and made every excuse to avoid his office. He lost fifteen pounds, quit talking to his wife, stopped walking his dog, wouldn't accept dinner invitations even though they were important to his wife, stared into space for hours on end, and let the grass and weeds grow and grow.

All the while, thousands of emails were coming into *The Times-Picayune* in response to Rose's columns about post-Katrina and its victims—"each of them little histories that would break your heart," he recalls. During months of driving through what looked like bombed-out neighborhoods, which were the grist for his news columns, he "met legions of people who appeared to be dying from sadness" and wrote about them. The city of New Orleans was traumatized. His readers resonated with his words.

But things were not getting better for Rose. After slogging through winter and spring, he ground to a halt by summer. "I was a dead man walking," he writes. "I had never been so scared in my life."

When you have been traumatized in the way that happened to the people of New Orleans, it's as if it were a life sentence. This is what Rose had begun to believe. He recollects, "I'm not going to get better, I thought. I'm in too deep."

One year after Katrina, Rose found relief when he began taking medication. The dark curtain lifted. He came to life again.

To take medication ran against Rose's lifelong philosophy of self-determination, but he finally realized he had a chemical imbalance. Medication became a necessary step to restore his ability to function. "My brain was literally shorting out," he writes. "The cells were not properly communicating. Chemistry imbalances, likely caused by increased stress hormones, were dogging the work of my neurotransmitters, my electrical wiring. A real and true physiological deterioration had begun."

A LIFE SENTENCE?

Here's a story of one of Rose's readers, caught in the emotional aftermath of Hurricane Katrina. It's a classic example of how, even in the world's wealthiest nation, with the greatest number of health professionals, an individual can begin to believe they will *always* suffer the effects of trauma, without hope of relief.

In this reader's case, it proved difficult to get sustenance into his stomach, as he watched himself shed pound after pound. His entire system was in a state of acute acidosis—so much so that he felt as though his stomach and esophagus were on fire most of the day.

As the months went by, the man found himself enduring continual anxiety and dread. Medication made him feel worse, even suicidal. He began to believe he was marked for life—that some irrevocable change had occurred in his body chemistry.

At a workshop one day, the individual's fears were confirmed by a therapist who explained that what he was experiencing was neither unique to him nor confined to a small number of the population. The condition was rampant in New Orleans and along the Gulf Coast. Suicide rates were sky-high, depression rife. "I can teach you techniques to manage your distress, but you will likely never be free of it," the workshop leader opined. "As part of coming to terms with this disaster, you need to accept that what has occurred will rob you of at least ten years of your life."

The therapist went on to explain, "If only we had been able to get you help in the first couple of weeks, you might have been spared the permanent effects of this trauma." The words felt like a death sentence. The individual began to reconcile himself to the idea that he would simply have to endure the agonizing stew of disturbing emotions he was experiencing without hope of them subsiding.

WHEN A PROFESSIONAL ISN'T AVAILABLE

Many who have been traumatized have sought help through medicine. But drug treatment is expensive, can have serious long-term side effects, and isn't readily available in all parts of the world.

As with medication, talk therapy isn't a possibility for everyone, either. Many cannot afford such a luxury. It also requires setting time aside each week to visit a particular location for treatment, often over an extended period. Even in Western nations, let alone the Third World, this is impractical for many—especially for those who work or have little children who are dependent on them. It can be difficult, if not impossible, for such individuals to free themselves to engage in long-term therapy.

Talk therapy becomes even more impractical and virtually impossible when large-scale disasters such as a tsunami, tornado, or earthquake traumatize thousands of people within a specific region in a matter of moments.

When we can find neither the time nor the money to see a therapist, or help isn't available because of where we live, what are we to do?

A WINDOW OPENS

One afternoon in the remote town of Dembidolo, Ethiopia, I took a break from the workshop I was giving and visited a Catholic church across the street.

Sitting in this mud sanctuary, lit only by a few rays of sun that managed to creep through the door and windows, my attention was drawn to an old man who entered the church, walked past me, and knelt on the dirt floor a few rows in front of me. The cotton shirt he was wearing was worn so thin you could see right through to his skin. As he knelt, the bottoms of his bare feet were exposed. Because of the red clay of the land and the dim lighting, I couldn't see where his feet ended and the clay began. Immediately the image of God making humans out of the clay of the earth came to mind.

As I continued to watch this humble man pray, I couldn't help but believe that if trauma can occur to every human being, then *a healing process must be available to everyone too.* For there was no way a man like this could ever afford professional counseling or medication.

This experience, coupled with my exposure to the poor, uneducated, and desperate war refugees to whom I was giving the workshop, forced me to question whether traditional therapy and long-term medication are truly the only way forward for a trauma victim.

Is it really the case that the effects of trauma can never be cured, but can only be managed with the help of professional counseling and drugs? Is the depression triggered by trauma inevitably a life sentence? Or is there an obvious natural solution—available to anyone, anywhere in the world—that we have overlooked, that can open the door that has locked us in our own isolation?

3

"Help Me Heal Myself"

❀ ❀ ❀ ❀ ❀

WE ARE LIVING IN AN ERA that holds the possibility of far more mass trauma than we have so far experienced in human history, due to the proliferation of terrorism and unresolved political crises in many nations—not to mention climate change, which is causing increased loss of life and habitat in the wake of more serious droughts, fires, floods, and hurricanes.

Tragic experiences seem to be escalating everywhere, so much so that trauma is being called "The Invisible Epidemic."[1]

From Hurricane Katrina to the tsunami in the Indian Ocean, and from genocide in Africa to suicide bombings in Iraq, the demand for assistance with trauma recovery is overwhelming. Added to this, since World War II there have been 250 wars resulting in the deaths of 30 million people, ninety percent of them civilians. Witness the wars in Iraq and Afghanistan, together with the violence in Pakistan, Burma, the Middle East, and other regions of the world. How do we as individuals, as nations, and as a global community hope to care for and resolve the traumatic experiences of such large populations?

Mainstream health care providers are finding they are unprepared for much of the trauma occurring on the planet. Lacking the required knowledge and training, they are often ill equipped to deal adequately with this large-scale crisis. There are simply not enough counselors, therapists, and medical practitioners to attend to the overwhelming suffering at this time in history.

Given the immensity of the crisis, we are in need of a new approach that can address trauma on both the individual and collective levels— and in multicultural settings. But what might such an approach be?

CLUES FROM AN ANCIENT PEOPLE

While working in Ethiopia, I discovered it's a common custom in the villages I visited for several families who live close to each other to have coffee together each morning. The ritual takes about two hours. They begin by roasting the beans, grinding them, then finally boiling them to make a fresh pot of coffee. During these two hours, they process what happened in their lives the day before.

Because the Ethiopian people I visited were living in a war zone, it was usual for them to discuss the tragedies they had personally experienced or heard about from others. As they shared their pain with each other, they also received encouragement.

The point of relating this experience isn't how effective these people were in processing their trauma, as if they had found the best way of dealing with what they were experiencing. Indeed, we shall see that talk therapy alone often isn't enough—especially once trauma is etched deeply into the body. The point is these Ethiopians were taking personal responsibility for their state of being. The people of this war-torn land had developed a natural form of dealing with the trauma they were experiencing, coping with it among themselves each day *as it occurred*.

These people didn't need individual sessions of private therapy with a skilled practitioner because the help they required was embedded in their cultural tradition. It wasn't necessary for them to understand Western psychological principles in order to process their experiences. They simply knew about pain, suffering, and being alongside each other to process what they were experiencing as they went through traumatic times.

In our more individualized culture, in which families have become nuclear and where close community connection has largely broken down, we no longer share extended periods of time together on a daily basis. For this reason, we feel a need to seek out professionals to help us resolve our pain. But could it be we have something to learn from the many cultures that have developed their own grassroots communal healing strategies? Historically, this is how humans have dealt with painful circumstances—by taking personal responsibility.

A CRY FOR HELP

Whatever trauma we may have experienced, even professional help is most effective when it empowers us to take our recovery into *our own hands*.

Professional counseling should always have a goal of enabling individuals to heal themselves. Along with giving them the skills to recover from their trauma, it must help individuals prepare for future times of trauma. This not only prevents therapy from becoming a form of dependency, the self-empowerment equips us with the necessary integrity to resolve our pain *ourselves*.

To the degree that it is viable and safe, trauma recovery must be taken out of the professional therapeutic domain and brought right into the household. The treatment needs to be capable of being self-applied, have rapid results, and be easy to use by large populations without the guidance of a therapist.

It's so obvious this is needed. As a client once told me out of desperation, "For two hours a week, I have your support during my healing process. For the remaining 166 hours in a week, I have to heal myself. Please give me something that I can do to help myself when you are not around!"

DESIGNED TO HANDLE TRAUMA

As I have traveled the world, I have come to understand that we humans possess an organic restorative capacity within our own body. Trauma doesn't have to mark us for life. In fact, *we can recover completely.*

Through my experience of working with traumatized Ethiopians, Eritreans, Sudanese, Americans, Israelis, Palestinians, and others—in situations of war, famine, and natural disasters—I have learned that no matter what our culture, language, religion, or psycho-social background, as traumatized individuals we have access to a natural process genetically encoded within the body that enables us to heal from trauma. The human body is capable of healing itself from even the most debilitating experiences. But it takes more than just time. It takes being aware of the body's restorative ability and actively encouraging it to do its work.

Because of the body's innate capacity to restore itself, I have come to believe that the healing of trauma can occur anywhere—in the midst of Western society or among whole populations in the most remote and destitute regions of the world. Not only is it possible to recover from terrible events that shock us almost to death, but through the process of recovering from trauma, we have the potential of becoming more ethical and caring people than we were capable of being prior to the traumatic event. If the recovery process is taken up in a serious manner, we will inevitably live a more productive and fulfilling life—in most cases without the cost of expensive prescription medicines and often without professional help.

BEYOND "TALKING IT OUT"

As living organisms, our bodies know we are capable of enduring and recovering from even the most severe of tragedies. To exist and evolve, we have developed an instinctual mechanism that enables us to let go of the past and begin something new. In fact, we are *compelled* physiologically to rid ourselves of anything that obstructs our survival. This way we can complete one phase of our life and begin the next.

Our fear of exploring the effects of trauma is a resistance to our natural evolutionary impulse. This resistance constrains our life force and inhibits our ability to grow internally, transform ourselves, and incorporate past experiences into our present life. Unless we let go of this resistance, we cannot replace the shattered structure of our sense of self with a healthy one.

Friedrich Nietzsche saw this. In *Untimely Meditations*, he says we possess "the power to grow uniquely from within, to transform and incorporate the past and the unknown, to heal wounds, to replace what is lost, and to duplicate shattered structures from within."[2]

This realization that we are designed to learn from and move beyond trauma led me to study the human body and design a method of trauma recovery that anyone in the world can follow. The approach to trauma recovery explained in this book is to empower us to take recovery from emotional pain into our own hands. For us to accomplish this, it's necessary to first understand what happens in our body when trauma befalls us.

4

When Life Doesn't Work Out the Way It's Supposed To

❁ ❁ ❁ ❁ ❁

WE SUDDENLY FIND OURSELVES in emotional distress, and we don't understand what's going on. It might even seem as if our life is spinning out of control. Nothing is working the way we think it's supposed to, and yet there is nothing life-threatening going on around us.

What's happening is that something in the present has triggered unprocessed trauma from the past, and this is now emerging as distress.

Consider the case of a woman in her thirties who was in bed one night with a man she was getting to know and trust. Usually the couple enjoyed intimacy in reduced lighting. But this particular night, the room was pitch black. As they moved toward intimacy, the woman suddenly leapt out of bed, ran from the room, and spent the next couple of hours on the phone with her sister.

When she returned to bed, the woman explained what had happened to her. She hadn't been in a particularly passionate frame of mind as they retired that night, but she nevertheless allowed herself to respond to her lover's advances. Suddenly, lying there in the dark, with her heart not really in what she was about to do, she experienced an overwhelming sense of panic.

This young woman had never discussed her sad relationship with her father with anyone. But that night, on the phone with her sister, she confirmed what she had long suspected—that her father had repeatedly come to her bed when she was a young girl. Equally distressing, her mother was aware that her daughter was being sexually abused and did nothing about it.

In the darkness, with this man she was becoming fond of, the young woman had suffered a vivid flashback to the times her father forced himself on her, which set off all her emotional alarms. She was in great distress.

GETTING INSIDE OUR HEAD

From the moment we were born, we have been receiving physical stimuli from the world around us. Some of this has been pleasant and some of it unpleasant. But all of it affects the quality of our life.

Those parts of our brain that receive input from our physical senses process millions of bits of data from the external world each and every day. When this information is welcome and not in any way distressing, our brain sends it to those areas associated with memories and feelings, which connect it to similar experiences from our past. In turn, this information is then passed to another area of the brain where it's turned into a story about our experience. This is how we make sense of the things that happen to us.

Consider what usually occurs when we meet someone for the first time. We shake hands. Does the person's handshake feel safe? Do they smile and make eye contact? If so, is the smile authentic, and does the person truly connect through the eyes? Our somatosensory brain (the word *soma* means "body") is taking all of this in—the sensation of the handshake, the smile, the eye contact.

When the information is transferred to the association area of the brain, it gets attached to memories of similar encounters. Next, the gnostic area of the brain puts together a story from all of this data and the associations it awakens. It begins to form a picture, which may say that the individual we just encountered is a nice person. If so, we are at ease about our meeting.

HOW THE BRAIN PROCESSES TRAUMA

Traumatic experiences are processed differently from pleasant sensations. Because these experiences are intrusive and result in an overwhelming arousal of our system, they are taken in as fragments rather than as a whole experience.

When data is taken in as fragments, it's stored in the sensory parts of the brain, where it remains compartmentalized. The trouble is, this area of the brain now has billions of bits of data that need to be associated with feelings, memories, and emotions, then sent to the gnostic area to be told as a story. As long as these bits of data are trapped in the sensory part of the brain, they remain chaotic and unhealed.

Years later, when life presents us with cues that closely match the unprocessed stimuli from a traumatic event, it tends to trigger these unintegrated memories, bringing them back to mind as if the event were occurring in the present. These stored and unprocessed sensations are what cause flashbacks and nightmares. It's as if the trauma were happening all over again.

For example, if we are in a car accident and there is a strong odor of leaking gas, we may not be aware of the odor during the accident because our ability to discern everything that's happening at such a moment is running on overload. But the next time we pull into a gas station, we have a flashback to the accident, triggering a measure of fear, and perhaps causing us to tremble—even though we are simply pumping gas. The odor of gas is being sent from the sensory area of the brain to the association area.

When such a flashback occurs, it can be helpful if we tell someone close to us about the incident. As we feel their support while we allow ourselves to experience our emotions, the emotions connected with the incident can be integrated if we are serious about healing and not simply wallowing in telling our story. In this way we are able to heal the traumatic memory, just as the people in the war zone I visited in Ethiopia were able to do over their morning coffee. The experience doesn't become lodged in our psyche or body.

TRAUMA CAN WRECK YOUR HEALTH

In addition to causing us emotional distress, unresolved trauma lies at the root of much chronic pain for which a cause has never been determined. It's also responsible for a host of common physical illnesses.

Thankfully, we now have direct evidence that when the traumatized state of an individual is corrected, physical symptoms tend to lessen considerably. In many cases they can go into remission, or even disappear for good. What facilitates these amazing changes in the body?

The autonomic nervous system, the endocrine system, and the immune system, which function in harmony, are all disrupted by trauma. In order to understand trauma's effects on the body, it's helpful to understand how these systems are disrupted.

Humans have different kinds of memory involving different aspects of the brain. The majority of what we learn, in the form of facts, together with most of the events we experience and the conversations we have with people, tend to be forgotten rather easily. The type of memory that retains such information is not only fragile but also subject to distortion by our emotions. This is why two people remember events, or what was said, differently.

In contrast, there are memories that become hardwired into the brain. When something triggers strong emotions, such as the planes crashing into the Twin Towers, the event is ingrained in us. We remember exactly where we were at the time and what we were doing.

Another form of memory, known as procedural memory, also involves hardwiring the brain. We use this type of memory to learn habits and skills when we are infants. For instance, it's how we learn to walk, ride a bicycle, play an instrument, or gain proficiency in a career skill.

In addition to retaining habits and skills, procedural memory is the aspect of our memory that can be conditioned to respond to specific cues of the kind the young woman in bed experienced, or that a person might experience at a gas station following an automobile accident. This part of our memory works in the same way a dog can be trained to salivate at the sound of a bell. This is because procedural memory stores the cues associated with the event—the smell, feel, taste, and images.

HOW ILLNESS RESULTS FROM TRAUMA

Trauma that we don't process close to the time of its occurrence causes a variety of secondary problems. Not only is the production of growth hormones, reproductive hormones, and digestion disrupted, but our emotions are not processed well either because our cognitive capacity is reduced. Prolonged stress also causes exhaustion of the adrenal glands, which has a profound inhibitory effect on our immune system.

There is now evidence that even excessive stress, let alone severe trauma, is a factor in a variety of illnesses. These include anxiety disorders, depression, high blood pressure, cardiovascular disease, gastrointestinal troubles, some cancers, and premature aging. Stress also seems to increase the frequency and severity of migraine headaches, episodes of asthma, and fluctuation of blood sugar in diabetics. Additionally, there is evidence that people experiencing significant psychological stress are more prone to develop colds and other infections than those who are less stressed. This is because stress reduces the efficiency of our immune system, which would normally fight off infection.

In addition to these adverse health effects, we have the ability to split off from normal consciousness those regions of the body through which trauma enters our lives. We dissociate ourselves from such a body part—literally shut it down, restricting circulation in this part of the body. We do this because the messages coming from this area of the body are perceived as a threat.

A muscle deprived of blood goes into spasm, which is extremely painful. With cues, the symptom occurs again, just as if the trauma itself were happening all over again. Muscles that became clenched in an act of self-defense during the original trauma replicate this clenching. In fact, as many as half of all symptoms for which people see doctors stem from this kind of clenching.

As an example, we can see how this works in terms of a woman's enjoyment of sex. The piriformis muscle in the buttock connects the thighbones to the pelvis and forms a cup in the posterior part of the pelvis, adjacent to the vagina. When this muscle is tense, it results in painful intercourse. This is especially prevalent when there has been sexual trauma such as rape, incest, or sodomy. The pain is being triggered by procedural memory, which causes one of the Kegel muscles to clench in an act of self-defense during a sexual assault. Intercourse "cues" the brain to remember the original trauma. This can also be one cause of sciatica.

In both males and females, pain can also develop in an extremity that is overused over a period of time, especially in the dominant hand, and hence is prevalent in people who use a keyboard and mouse continuously. If a person lives in a state of arousal as a result of previous trauma, repetitive contraction of an already contracted muscle can cause the muscle to become inflamed. This can produce a variety of symptoms such as carpal tunnel syndrome, impingement syndrome in the shoulder, cervical disc disease in the neck, TMJ, and migraine.

Tics might occur based on old traumatic events that were never resolved. Not without reason do we call them nervous tics. Other habitual spasms might include a squinting eye and throat-clearing.

A cluster of diseases may be associated with the way people often freeze in the face of danger. Gut and chest-related symptoms include irritable bowel syndrome, constipation, cramps and diarrhea, and gastro-esophageal reflux. There is some evidence to suggest that fibromyalgia and chronic fatigue syndrome may also be connected with the freeze response, as well as phantom limb pain following an amputation.

Multiple chemical sensitivity can often be triggered by a smell such as new carpet, cigarette smoke, or perfume. The person has become progressively sensitive, until the slightest threat triggers autonomic dysregulation. Although migraines can be genetic, they can also occur as a result of the dilating and constriction of blood vessels. Asthma, too, results from constriction in the lungs that may be connected with trauma. A stutter, premenstrual syndrome, and postpartum psychosis can be exacerbated by trauma. Attention deficit hyperactivity disorder and sleep apnea can also be related to trauma.

Though trauma causes a plethora of physical symptoms, many of these abate when we create a psychophysical climate that *allows the body to heal itself*. How we can create such a climate will become clear once we have a thorough understanding of how trauma is experienced in the body.

5

How Our Instant-on Button Gets Stuck

❀ ❀ ❀ ❀ ❀

PSYCHOLOGY ORIGINALLY FOCUSED on the ego and unconscious as the source of anxiety and stress, which meant anxiety and stress were considered a product of social conditioning. On the other hand, neurologists have followed a trail that leads to the interaction of certain parts of the brain as the source of emotion, while physiologists focused on the role of the nervous system in stress and anxiety. Yet another group of researchers—psychobiologists—focused on the neuropeptides and other chemicals generated in the brain and transmitted throughout the body as a major contributor to stress and anxiety.

It's been said that all roads lead to Rome. Similarly, it's becoming increasingly clear that these different routes of research into how we experience stress, anxiety, and trauma are leading us to the recognition that body and mind are intricately linked. The reaction we have to trauma results from an exquisite mutual interdependence between the body's different systems, which work together toward the single objective of ensuring our survival.

Medically speaking, the physiological reactions we experience in response to stress are quite distinct from the psychological state known as anxiety. Yet it's through the intricate interaction of these different systems that anxiety is generated. When these psycho-biological-neurological changes occur, they trigger an increase in both our heart rate and our blood pressure. This results in the uncomfortable sensation we describe as anxiety. This physiological change now affects us psychologically, as we register the discomfort caused by these stress changes. We then give a psychological interpretation to what we are feeling physically. Anxiety is therefore both physiological and psychological.

A PROTECTIVE SYSTEM GONE AWRY

Humans have an instant-on button that protects us by causing us either to fight, flee, or freeze when a threat to our survival looms.

The hypothalamus-pituitary-adrenal axis (known as HPA) is a system that links the limbic system of the brain with the adrenal glands. The limbic system of the brain is the control center for most of the body's hormonal functions. The hypothalamus and pituitary glands, as well as the amygdala, reside here. Directly connected to the adrenal glands that are located on top of the kidneys, the hypothalamus and pituitary glands produce hormones in response to any type of physical or psychological stress. Because this is an aspect of the brain that humans and all other mammals have in common with reptiles, it's sometimes referred to as the "reptilian brain."

In times of trauma, the hypothalamus-pituitary-adrenal axis is activated and produces neurotransmitters. These are hormones that function as chemical messengers, the likes of dopamine, norepinephrine, and epinephrine (more commonly known as adrenaline). When we detect a potentially threatening situation, the body produces these chemicals to reinforce our ability to defend ourselves.

Simultaneously, under normal circumstances, the sympathetic nervous system and the parasympathetic nervous system, which together make up the autonomic nervous system, are primed. They work to help us survive by maintaining a steady state throughout our many complex bodily systems, which would otherwise go haywire in the face of trauma.

The systems that take charge during an emergency suspend all unnecessary bodily functions and activate only those essential for survival. With the fight-flight response, we can experience a variety of sensations such as arousal, anxiety, panic, phobias, bracing our muscles, tremors, high blood pressure, rapid heartbeat, and tachycardia. Our mouth can become dry, our hands cold. Although our growth hormones, reproductive hormones, and digestion are essential in normal everyday life, their functioning can be suspended in an emergency.

The trouble is, a protective response to stress that serves us for a short time can cause serious long-term harm if the stress is unabated.

STUCK IN THE PAST

In the normal course of events, the hypothalamus-pituitary-adrenal axis is deactivated after a stressful occurrence has passed. The parasympathetic nervous system then becomes dominant again, and the individual returns to a relaxed state.

The dilemma of the human species is that although thoughts can easily trigger anxiety by activating the hypothalamus-pituitary-adrenal axis, we're not as effective at turning it off. Our instant-on button can become stuck, so that we can't readily extinguish anxiety after a traumatic event.

Once we are in a stuck mode, the effects of trauma become long lasting. Our inability to extinguish the activity of our hypothalamus-pituitary-adrenal axis is why we continue feeling anxious years after a stressful event is over. Even when we try to remain calm, the unconscious running of the limbic system causes us to feel anxious.

Anxiety is unresolved fear. It's a feeling of disquiet, marked by dread and foreboding. Prolonged anxiety can manifest disorders such as panic attacks, social phobias, and post-traumatic stress disorder. All of these conditions reflect a single underlying response of the limbic system. But whereas stress usually resolves itself after the stressful event has passed, in the case of prolonged anxiety, the symptoms persist.

RESURRECTING THE PAST

It doesn't matter how long ago a trauma occurred, the body always seeks to free us of its effects. It has a natural tendency toward healing that we can learn to work with once we are aware of it.

Even when, years later, an event triggers pain from our past, this pain is not without purpose. Though we believe that time heals wounds, and that we simply "get beyond" painful episodes, this isn't necessarily so.

Trauma, when unhealed, will sooner or later surface into our awareness again—something a young mother discovered years after her children were grown. "As I write this," she confided, "tears are streaming down my face, and my throat is knotted up as I relive, as if it were yesterday, the emotional trauma I suffered during the time my baby was in daycare and I was working. Maybe this had something to do with the gift his birth gave me. After about three months, I reached the depths of my suffering. I was sitting at my desk one day with what seemed like an eternity before I would see my baby, saying to myself, 'I can't take this anymore! I can't stand to be away from him like this! Another woman holds my sweet little angel more than I do! I have to work, but I can't do this any longer! Please God, please! Help me!' I had no idea this wound was still so wide open."

This mother had simply stuffed her feelings deep inside her because she lacked the knowledge of how to process the trauma she was going through.

One of the miracles of brain functioning is that as we pass through the various stages of maturation—adolescence, mid-life, and our later wisdom years—our brain automatically tries to rid itself of unresolved sensory memories. At appropriate moments, it spontaneously sends these memories to the association area.

This mother is like so many people who, approaching midlife, find themselves remembering traumatic childhood experiences—particularly sexual abuse. That such issues should arise seemingly out of nowhere can be frightening. But nothing is going wrong. On the contrary, by bringing unresolved issues to our attention at this time in our life, the brain is serving us well. It's attempting to rid itself of unnecessary baggage so it can prepare for the new stimuli it will experience in its next stage of development.

6

Beyond the Therapist's Couch

❀ ❀ ❀ ❀ ❀

THE EMOTIONAL PAIN WE CARRY within us isn't just in our head. It's also etched into our muscles.

When I was living in Lebanon during a period of severe fighting, I inadvertently found myself in a section of the city controlled by warring factions that prevented any civilians from escaping. I sought refuge in an abandoned, bombed-out school building, living for several weeks in the basement of this building with seven other people.

Our only means of obtaining food was from a tank driver who knew we were trapped in the building. Each day when he patrolled the streets, he searched out abandoned stores from which to gather supplies, delivering them to us in his tank at the end of the day.

One day there was particularly intense fighting with tanks and mortar shells. The battle lasted the entire day, and the eight of us who were caught in this building spent the day in the basement sitting on the floor with our backs against the wall and our knees bent in a semi-fetal position. During the shelling, many mortars hit the three-story structure. Each time a shell landed, the entire edifice shuddered as the sound of the explosion boomeranged through the building.

No matter how accustomed we became to the explosions, each shock-wave *instinctively caused us to jerk into the fetal position*. There was nothing conscious about this reaction. It was an automatic response to the intensity of the loud explosions.

During one mortar hit, I happened to be watching my trapped colleagues, talking to them as they sat helplessly against the wall. As the shell exploded, I was stunned by what I observed. Every single one of us was startled, then instantly contracted in an identical way. It was as though I were watching a well-rehearsed piece of choreography.

Although we had been doing this all day, it was only now that I realized how precise our response was. From the moment of being startled, to moving into a tight fetal position, our movements were perfectly coordinated.

I knew I had stumbled onto something that was completely obvious—so obvious that I hadn't paid attention to it until now. Each of us had been enacting a pattern of behavior that was neither accidental nor random.

But why did the body make this particular movement? Why not some other kind of movement, or a variety of different movements? My curiosity was awakened. How did all of us know to make the exact same movements in unison and with such precision?

The eight of us were from six different countries, so this meant that our movements were not culturally determined. They had to spring from a source that was deeper and more primitive within all humans.

THE WISDOM OF THE BODY

The incident in the school basement was the first time I realized the body has a genetically encoded response that's designed to protect us. It's a primal response found in all humans, performed spontaneously whenever we are endangered.

As a massage therapist, I was interested in exploring which specific set of muscles is used to accomplish this movement. How are the brain and body organized to facilitate this particular behavior?

When I departed from Lebanon months later, I studied the anatomy of the body to determine which muscles generated this movement. With the help of a neurologist, I learned that humans, like other mammals, have an instinctual memory of what we need to do when we are endangered. The brain unhesitatingly triggers body movements to increase our chances of survival when we are at risk of bodily harm.

Initially, the brain perceives something as threatening, whereupon it instructs certain organs to produce the chemicals required to survive the danger. These chemicals are then pumped into the muscles of the body to provide the necessary protection.

The response of muscles exposed to stressful events is to contract. During any traumatic experience, the body performs this process by contracting the flexor muscles located in the anterior of the body. When these contract, they inhibit the extensor muscles located in the posterior of the body. This creates what is known as flexor withdrawal.

The combination of flexor contraction and extensor relaxation allows the body to bring our extremities together, "creating a fetal-like enclosure that causes us to feel safer by protecting our vulnerable soft parts—our genitals, vital organs, and the head with its eyes, ears, nose, and mouth."[3]

Two of the primary flexor muscles that contract to protect the underbelly of the human animal are the psoas muscles. These primitive muscles stand guard like sentinels protecting the center of gravity of the human body, located just in front of the third vertebrae of the sacrum. The psoas muscles connect the back with the pelvis and the legs. They are the only muscles that do this. They also connect with all five lumbar vertebrae.

The protective procedure, stored deep in the brain, automatically springs into action to contract these muscles when we are threatened, spontaneously taking us through the steps we need to go through to contract the body for our safety.

When the psoas muscles contract and pull the body forward, they cause secondary muscle contractions as the body tries to compensate for this forward pull. At the same time, the erector spinae muscles pull the body backwards in an attempt to keep it upright. These two opposing tensions pull the lower vertebrae together, creating a spinal compression. This can be damaging if the compression is prolonged. Indeed, if the tension is continued long enough, it will eventually cause shoulder and neck pain as well. To heal from trauma contractions, this deep set of muscles must let go of their tension and relax.

It's generally accepted that after a particularly tense, stressing, or traumatic experience, we can simply get a massage, take a hot bath, do some exercise, and this will restore our body to a healthy state. But when it comes to traumatic tension in the psoas muscles, this isn't the case. Contracted or damaged psoas muscles can cause severe and persistent lower back pain. This is especially common among sexual abuse survivors.

Because the reaction of the human body during trauma alters the tone of our skeletal muscles and their ability to function, if these changes in our muscles go unreleased, they will develop into patterns of chronic tension that will eventually create additional bodily dysfunction. Unless they are returned to a relaxed state after the stressful event is over, they are particularly vulnerable to continued stimulation, causing us to react to even minor stress with anxiety.

It's vital to be able to turn off this muscular response to stress.

IT TAKES MORE THAN TRADITIONAL COUNSELING

The field of psychology has made a considerable contribution to our understanding of the psyche. However, as science has advanced, we have realized that psychological approaches to trauma recovery, though helpful, are limited in what they can accomplish. This is because psychology deals with the content of the mind.

Neurology, on the other hand, deals with the way the brain processes this content. For successful trauma recovery, it's necessary to deal with the content of the brain, the manner in which the brain processes the content, and the physical and spiritual changes the person experiences in the recovery process.

In short, recovery from trauma requires attention to the body, mind, and spirit at different stages of the recovery process. None of these dimensions of the human person can be overlooked in the recovery process.

New research is beginning to recognize that the body is more involved in the traumatic experience than previously understood. Thus physical techniques are beginning to surface that can produce brain balance by shutting down the amygdala and allowing the traumatic cues trapped in the brain to trickle to the surface like bubbles escaping from a bottle of carbonated water.

These new body techniques help the brain to shift into a state of empowerment, whereby it is no longer ruled by past cues but functions in the present moment. An empowered person doesn't feel helpless. We no longer live with traumatic cues interrupting our day and making our lives unpleasant.

BRINGING THE BODY INTO THE PICTURE

A variety of stress reduction techniques attempt to interrupt the continuing activity of the hypothalamus-pituitary-adrenal axis. One of the most promising is physical exercise.

Research on exercise for the improvement of mental health is not new. In fact, considerable research has been conducted on the effects of exercise on a variety of common human experiences. As a result, we know that exercise lowers stress levels as well as reduces anxiety. It has also been shown to be beneficial for everything from enhancing self-esteem to improving sleep. Indeed, its use to help relieve stress, anxiety, and even depression—while enhancing mood, self-esteem, and body image—has a long history.

Depression can be debilitating. But as early as 1905, research suggested exercise has a positive effect on this condition. Since that time, major studies of the effect of exercise on depression have shown promising results. Exercise has an antidepressant effect on the body because it creates the stimulants norepinephrine, dopamine, and serotonin, which are natural antidepressants. The benefits of exercise may be detected as early as the first session and generally continue beyond the end of the exercise program.

Aerobic exercises focus on endurance, intensity, and resistance. Although aerobic exercise has shown a positive correlation to reduced stress, anxiety, and depression, it hasn't been clear whether there is an exercise routine that's particularly useful for addressing emotional trauma.

GETTING AT THE MUSCLES

Alongside the kind of therapy in which we talk about our issues, a whole raft of therapies known as psychosomatic therapies recognize that the pain we seek to express by talking is actually trapped in our physical makeup.

Psychosomatic approaches to counseling arose during the 20th century because of the limitations of talk therapy, and a variety of therapies now combine both psychotherapy and body therapy in the same session. In fact, there is now a long history of therapies that employ direct physical attempts to release trapped energy. These include Orgone Therapy developed by Wilhelm Reich in the 1940s, Bioenergetic Analysis developed by Alexander Lowen in the 1950s, Core Energetics developed by John C. Pierrakos in the 1970s, Holotropic Breathwork developed by Stanislav Grof also in the 1970s, Thought Field Therapy developed by Roger J. Callahan in the 1980s, and Eye Movement Desensitization and Reprocessing developed by Francine Schapiro in the 1980s.

One factor common in all of these techniques is that they recognize *tremors* as an expression of an overactive sympathetic nervous system. People *shake* when they are traumatized. However, the purpose and potential therapeutic value of shaking has not been adequately explored.

7

How the Body Copes with Trauma

❀ ❀ ❀ ❀ ❀

I WAS LIVING IN A SMALL VILLAGE in Africa that was caught in the middle of severe fighting. This particular country had been at war for many years and the village experienced frequent aerial bombings. One afternoon, the men of the village were sitting around talking when the chickens and dogs began running about wildly. This alerted us that a plane was headed towards us. Whenever aircraft approached, it was the task of the adults to gather as many children as possible and run with them to the bomb shelters.

Once in the bomb shelters, which were quite small and primitive, the adults seated themselves on benches and held the children on their knees. During this particular bombing, I had two children in my care, each around two years of age. As bombs struck the ground, it felt as though the earth itself was shuddering. The closer the bombing came to the shelter, the stronger the shuddering became. It was a terrifying experience.

At one point, I realized that the children on my lap were shaking all over—much like a dog in a thunderstorm or a person experiencing extreme cold. Of course, I had felt this shaking on previous occasions, but this was the first time I questioned what purpose these body tremors served. Why were these children trembling?

Research suggests that tremors associated with some diseases may not be a symptom so much as they are self-induced by the body in an attempt to detoxify itself through increased metabolism and lymphatic circulation. But what about tremors produced in times of trauma?

TREMBLING WITH FRIGHT

Animals that live in their natural habitats often encounter trauma. Once the initial fight, flight, or freeze reaction is over, how do they process this trauma?

If a gazelle is attacked by a lion but manages to escape, its entire body will shiver for a while. This trembling is a way of shaking out the excess charge. After the adrenalin has been released, the gazelle returns to the herd, drinking water from the pond as though nothing had happened.[4]

If two waterfowl on a lake get into an altercation over territory, they swim apart following the encounter, flapping their wings vigorously to shake off the effects.

We can also observe trembling in our own pets at moments when they are afraid of thunder and lightening. Faced with a frightening event like this, they generate the energy needed for either fight or flight. But because they are not in the wild and can come close to us and feel our reassuring presence, they don't need this energy and the body tremors to dispel it.

As with many mammals, tremoring occurs naturally in humans when we are either shaken up or nervous. For instance, people often report uncontrollable shaking after a car accident or some other brush with danger. If we feel nervous, our jaw may quiver and our teeth chatter. A classic example is giving a speech, which for many is one of life's most intimidating experiences. At such a time, we may find our knees knocking. Even on happy occasions like a wedding, a bride or groom can become so nervous that they find their hands trembling. Similarly, if the boss calls us on the carpet, our cheeks may quiver, or we may find ourselves shaking all over. In fact, we often say, "I shook like a leaf." Some of us also tremble when the blue lights and siren of a police vehicle go on behind us. And have you ever felt so enraged that you literally shook with anger?

Tremors are found in many cultures. Although there are no precise estimates of their incidence and prevalence, they are so common that they are recognized as a diagnostic feature of panic attacks, social phobias, anxiety disorder, and post-traumatic stress disorder.

The shivers that occur during trauma in animals come on at a precise time in the recovery process. Could it be that humans, who are also mammals, also tremor after traumatic events at a precise time and for a specific reason?

TREMORING IS GOOD FOR US

Much the same as the instinctual tremors in animals, tremors in humans are the natural response of a shocked or disrupted nervous system attempting to restore the body and mind to a state of balance.

Tremors are able to aid recovery because they don't cause us to relive the experience and thereby compound the trauma. On the contrary, they extinguish the trauma by helping us turn off our fight, flight, or freeze mechanism. They also discharge the excess energy from an aborted fight-or-flight response.

Tremors allow an organism to "thaw out" from the hyper-arousal state. They are the way the body releases itself from trauma. They work by quieting the hypothalamus-pituitary-adrenal axis in humans just as they do in other mammals. The body evokes the tremors to complete the discharge of our fight, flight, or freeze response.

Such tremors are referred to as *neurogenic* tremors. They are a primordial bodily experience originating in the processes of the brain's procedural memory. As such, they are a natural aspect of the genetic composition of the human organism.

An important aspect of a successful recovery from trauma is to activate the organism's natural release mechanism that signals the body to return to a state of rest and recuperation.

In 1997, Dr. Peter Levine articulated not only the theory behind tremors but also a process to evoke these tremors in the context of counseling. Dr. Levine proposes that the key to restoring balance in humans following a traumatic experience lies in our ability to "mirror the fluid adaptation of wild animals as they 'shake out' and pass through the immobility response and become fully mobile and functional again."[5] He calls the process he devised to accomplish this Somatic Experiencing.[6] Somatic Experiencing achieves extinction of the aborted discharge.

IF YOU TREMBLE, ARE YOU OUT OF CONTROL?

I have described how, during an air raid on an African village caught in the crossfire of a war, I sat holding two children. As the raid continued, it struck me that *only* the children were trembling. Why were the adults not shaking too?

That afternoon, the realization came to me that I was tensing myself *against* my natural instinct to tremble. It actually felt as though my body wanted to experience the tremors the children were experiencing, but I either wouldn't or couldn't let it—I didn't know which. I just knew that if I let myself go, I would shake all over.

When the bombing was over, I casually mentioned to the adults present that I had noticed how the children all trembled, and that I too had felt like I wanted to tremble. Each confided that they also wanted to tremble, but they resisted because they didn't wish the children to know they were afraid.

This response was so consistent on the part of the adults, it testifies to what neurologists who have studied this phenomenon conclude—that we have been *socialized out of* our ability to discharge stress by trembling. Unlike children and mammals in the wild, we've suppressed this natural tremoring experience because we find it embarrassing.

Giving into trembling makes us feel that we are "out of control," so it is deemed socially unacceptable and to be avoided. When we see someone trembling, it makes us uncomfortable because we don't know what to do about it.

Earlier I cited the case of a woman who had been repeatedly sexually abused by her father. Once she connected her fear of sex in the dark with what happened to her at the hands of her father, even the thought that her new lover might "expect" her to have sex terrified her. She found herself uncontrollably and quite violently shaking—a phenomenon that so frightened her lover, the relationship ended. Of course, he had no idea that his girlfriend's body was using shaking as a tool for healing. For him, shaking like this meant there was something seriously psychologically wrong with the person.

It's well accepted in the medical literature that body tremors are present in a number of psychological illnesses. However, to read this literature, one could imagine that the only reason the body tremors is because an individual has a reduced ability to cope with stressful situations. Little attention is paid to the fact that tremoring occurs far more widely than in psychological illnesses and is in fact a natural phenomenon.

HOLDING IT IN

As a society, we don't find it acceptable to demonstrate signs of vulnerability. A quivering voice, shaking legs, knees, and hands are interpreted as weakness in our culture. Therefore, instead of giving into our natural inclination to tremble, we often anesthetize our pain with medicine, alcohol, or other sedating substances.

For example, a group of male friends were sitting around their vehicles just off the highway, when a car that was speeding by hit another car, flipped over, and came careening towards the group, who scattered to save their lives. As the car came to a stop upside down, the men ran towards it and managed to pull out the occupants and provide first aid until medical professionals arrived. The scene was bloody and chaotic.

Afterwards, I spoke with each of the men about their different reactions. All of them reported shaking, which they found both uncomfortable and embarrassing. To deal with this, one went to a local bar and downed several drinks, numbing his body to calm his nerves. Another went home and got into bed without talking about the incident—though two days later, when he was alone in the house, he began to shake uncontrollably. Two others were shaking so badly at the scene that the police offered to drive them home, where they continued to shake for several hours.

Trauma and tragedy often find their way into our lives despite our best attempts at protecting ourselves. As living organisms, our bodies know we are capable of experiencing, enduring, and recovering from even the most severe trauma. It's our ego—the image we carry in our head of who we are—that tries to avoid and deny our vulnerability, and this places body and mind in conflict. Our body wants to shake to discharge the excess energy, but our mind refuses to let it do so. Our mind usually wins, and our body then must find another way of dealing with this hyper-aroused charge.

As a result of the prevailing belief that tremors indicate something is wrong with us, the purpose and potential therapeutic value of these tremors has received little attention. Thankfully, this releasing mechanism is still very much alive in our bodies, simply waiting for us to reactivate it for our healing.

It's time for us to recognize that shaking is a healthy function that has a physiological rather than a psychological origin. The activation and deactivation of the hypothalamus-pituitary-adrenal axis isn't a cultural or social phenomenon, but a natural physical process. By reinforcing and harnessing these primordial and instinctual tremors instead of treating them as if they were pathological, we are able to resolve the bodily manifestations of the overactive state of our sympathetic nervous system, restoring a state of balance.

After an incident of trauma is over, our nervous system should naturally deactivate itself by shaking out any residual tension-causing chemicals remaining from the traumatic episode. This shaking sends a signal to the brain informing it that the danger has subsided, and it should turn off its alert status.

If the nervous system doesn't deactivate itself, the body continues to remain in a kind of short-circuited loop, with our brain continuing to believe it's still in danger and therefore commanding the body to maintain a state of readiness. Consequently, our muscles hold onto the excess charge. If they don't get an opportunity to release this charge, they create a chronic tension pattern within the body.

When the flexor muscles don't return to a relaxed state after the stressful event is over, they also remain vulnerable to continued stimulation from even minor amounts of stress, setting up a vicious cycle of unending anxiety.

I wondered what would happen were I to deliberately relax this specific set of muscles that cause the movement towards the fetal position. I set out to find a way to cause these deep core muscles to relax.

TESTING THE THEORY

A student's life isn't as easy as it's often made out to be. This period of one's life that's sectioned off for learning, especially at the highly competitive college level, can be extremely stressful.

"I just don't know that I can maintain the 4.0 my parents expect of me," says a coed entering her junior year of college. "My philosophy professor has such high standards, it feels like it's impossible to get an A. If I don't make a 93 on that paper, I don't know how I'll tell my Dad."

On a quite different campus, a graduate student sighs, "It's make or break," as he enters a three-hour examination that will decide his career.

Elsewhere, a young woman who is submitting her doctoral thesis with its third set of amendments complains that the research requirements were so exacting, she's had to go on medication.

Each semester, term papers pile up in quick succession, stressing students to breaking point. Any escape from the study grind inevitably leads to regret. How do you juggle the demands of classes, study, working a job, and self-care, when you also need time for the socializing of college years that helps you keep your sanity?

Studies show that college students are experiencing increasing stress. On top of a heavy load of classes and work, they suffer from fear of evaluation by superiors, managing relationships with faculty members, and maintaining good peer relationships. As a result of the increasing levels of stress in this population, numerous research projects for stress reduction have been conducted among students.

I devised a study to test the physical and psychological effects of a unique exercise routine to reduce stress among this college population. The exercise routine doesn't involve the traditional aerobic components of endurance, intensity, or resistance. Instead, it focuses on eliciting body tremors.

The tremors are generated in the flexor muscles by performing a series of exercises that stretch the leg and pelvic muscles. The Trauma Release Process™ described in the second part of this book evokes our natural ability to shake ourselves back to a state of tranquility.

Herein lies the distinction between aerobic exercise for stress reduction and exercises that activate tremors. Aerobic exercise is under the direct control of the cortex—the part of the brain that gives us the ability to consciously control the body. So when we perform aerobic exercise, we can only do so to the extent that our mind allows. Also, we can only relax to the degree that our mind allows.

While there are yogis in the East who can slow their heart rate and lower their blood pressure consciously, in most of us this part of the brain isn't under our conscious control—that is, not readily influenced by the cerebral cortex, which is the seat of the will.

This is where tremors have the advantage. Because they are generated from within the limbic system of the brain, they are not under our conscious control. In other words, exercises that produce tremors bypass the thinking brain, giving us direct access to the unconscious reptilian brain. This enables us to bring about changes that we couldn't otherwise accomplish. By interrupting the hypothalamus-pituitary-adrenal axis, tremors produce physical relaxation, reducing our stress without need for our conscious control or even awareness of the releasing process.

ALL TENSED UP

A year after 9/11, it had become apparent to most people that the first responders—particularly police, fire personnel, and emergency medical teams—were still experiencing symptoms of post-traumatic stress disorder. These manifested themselves in different ways with different people. The exact symptoms have a lot to do with a person's disposition, the amount of healing support they receive, the closeness of their relationship to those who were killed, and their own childhood and adult experiences.

I was invited to New York by a group of therapists who had been working with post-traumatic stress disorder among the firefighters who were at Ground Zero. Their physical complaints included lower back pain, neck pain, shoulder pain, and gastro-intestinal problems. Having worked with the psoas muscles for years, I know that all of these symptoms can be the result of chronic contraction of the psoas.

I had the New York firefighters do the Trauma Release Process™ for two days. The first day, I explained the postures their bodies assumed and the movements they went through during their rescue efforts. These included bending forward, lifting, crawling, and being hunched down. The psoas muscle contracts tightly during these physical experiences. These positions are also emotionally charging, since they are accompanied by a fear of death. Consequently, the neural patterns established to hold the muscles in this tight position are also charged with a life-or-death intensity.

The Trauma Release Process™ helped these men and women to relax the contracted psoas muscle after only two sessions. The reason these exercises are so fast acting is that the tremors release the chronic tension from the inside of the muscle, rather than from the outside as in externally applied techniques such as massage.

It was an amazing experience to watch these firefighters release deep chronic tension simply by activating their tremoring mechanism. This mechanism did exactly what it's designed to do—restore the body to its natural state after a traumatic event.

Since they continue to put themselves in the path of danger daily, many firefighters do these exercises today as a regular part of their routine.

8

What Your Gut Instinct Is

❀ ❀ ❀ ❀ ❀

UNDER NORMAL CIRCUMSTANCES our brain takes in information, processes it through the emotions of the limbic system, and sends it to the neocortex for logical analysis and a reasonable response.

However, this process changes during a traumatic event. The individual must act quickly, which in most cases means instinctively. In order to do this, the brain utilizes its more primitive parts—the brain stem and limbic system. There is an immediate reaction, without the laborious and potentially dangerous process of reflection required for a logical response.

For example, soldiers are sitting around talking when suddenly a mortar shell hits close by. Everyone jumps up. Some dive for cover, while others run. None of these soldiers makes a conscious decision about what they end up doing. It's purely an instinctive response. Afterwards, they may even criticize one another or joke about their responses. But all of them will say, "I don't know why I reacted that way, I just did." The sudden threat of death causes the brain to respond according to its reptilian instinct. It simply reacts.

This process protects us during a time of danger. However, if we live in repeated or prolonged experiences of danger, we reinforce this reactive pattern—and the more we use this pattern, the more our brain will default to it even when we are no longer in danger. In other words, the more this neurological network is activated, the more this temporary state will develop into a permanent trait.

WHEN OBJECTIVITY IS IMPAIRED

In repeated or continual experiences of trauma, it's easy to become desensitized to the danger we are in. When this happens, our wellbeing is at risk. Sometimes it can even cost us our life.

A case in point comes from when I was working in a long-term counseling center. A missionary who was suffering from depression, anxiety, and extreme guilt came to work with me. She was part of a missionary group of women who had been working in an African country for years, and their presence among the local population was respected. But lately, the political atmosphere had become strained and extremist groups were springing up everywhere. Numerous outbursts of violence occurred, including kidnappings, bombings, and shootouts among the various factions.

My client was a close friend of the Superior for this group of women. The Superior had come from Europe to assess the severity of the situation. Shortly after her arrival, she recognized the danger that these women were living in. Voicing her concern to the women, she was assured by them that they were safe and wanted to continue their work. Against her instinct, the Superior agreed to let them stay, as long as they knew they must leave if the situation worsened. The Superior then returned to Europe.

Two weeks later a rebel group of insurgents broke into the women's home, accused them of being spies, and killed every last one of them. The distress around this incident was overwhelming. The Superior blamed herself for these deaths.

This is an example of how the neurological effects of trauma can cause impaired judgment, especially when the trauma is unrelenting. The brain—which should normally use the logic of the neocortex to make responsible decisions—becomes hijacked by the limbic system. Consequently, it makes irrational, emotional decisions. In this case, the women had been in a traumatic environment so long that their natural capacity for objectivity regarding their own safety had become obscured. They actually needed external help to make a responsible decision regarding their safety.

The Superior didn't realize that her observations of the danger these women were living in were more accurate than the women's own logic, which had been impaired. Had the Superior realized how trauma affects neural functioning, she could have explained the differences between their assessment of the situation and hers, possibly altering the decision of the group.

A more common example of this is someone who is in a car accident. Although not injured, the individual is too shaken to drive home. Even though they may try to assure us that they are physically okay, which they may be, their natural capacity for objectivity regarding their own safety and health has become obscured and they need external intervention in their decision-making.

THREE MUSKETEERS

We have discussed the role of the psoas muscles in trauma. The diaphragm muscle also adds to the tension in this area. As one researcher pointed out, "The attachments of the psoas muscle overlap those of the iliacus and diaphragm. Like the three musketeers, these muscles are 'one for all and all for one.' "[7] Together these muscles form a "muscular chain." This chain is the junction for the largest network of sympathetic nerves in the body—the solar plexus, often called the "abdominal brain." The abdominal-pelvic brain is a bundle of nerves located in the lower abdomen and pelvis. These nerve bundles contain more sympathetic nerves (fight-or-flight) than any other part of the body. This is where our gut feelings originate.

During trauma, the body places a priority on the abdominal-pelvic brain over the cranial brain. This is why people often begin to intuit danger prior to knowing that danger really does exist. The gut signals to the cranial brain to be on alert. Because we place such a high priority on the logic of the cranial brain, if there is no evidence to support the intuitive sensation of the gut, the cranial brain will override its sensations. This physiological process is what produces the inner doubt and questioning that we experience when there is no logical reason for our feelings, yet we are clearly experiencing sensations of danger.

Our society diminishes this sensory experience in everyday ordinary life, yet soldiers during a time of war are encouraged to be alert to any sensations of danger they experience, even if there is no data to confirm the danger.

As an example of how the gut works, a woman was walking down a dark street and sensed that something wasn't quite right. There were no obvious signs to confirm her intuition. In fact, everything seemed quite normal. Nevertheless, an inner dialogue began to take place between her gut, which is activated by sensation, and her cranial brain, which is activated by obvious signs. Despite the fact that our culture has discouraged women from relying on their intuition, and even diminishes them for doing so, her internal struggle intensified.

The woman told herself, "I'm making it up. There's nothing wrong." And yet she felt unsafe.

Just then, she saw a shadow of a figure coming out of an alley. Startled, she screamed. Fortunately, this chased the would-be attacker away. After the woman arrived home, she continued to debate within herself about why she didn't listen to her intuition. Her feelings were so strong, why didn't she respect them?

How many first responders must have felt danger in their gut as they entered the Twin Towers and yet went ahead anyway out of a sense of duty and dedication—only to lose their lives.

Culturally we are taught to disregard our gut instinct. But it is a crucial element of our ability to face and cope with traumatic situations.

9

Drowning in Trauma

❀ ❀ ❀ ❀ ❀

EARTH HAS AN EVER-INCREASING FAMILY of trauma survivors. We are most aware of trauma among people who are exposed to accidents or natural disasters such as earthquakes, tsunamis, hurricanes, tornadoes, droughts, floods, and fire. We are also aware of trauma among victims of war and political violence. Neither can we forget the many forms of societal trauma, such as community violence, aggravated assault, attempted kidnapping, and spousal and child abuse.

Individuals, certain communities, entire races such as Native Americans, and indeed whole nations have at times been "othered," and consequently experienced a disproportionate amount of trauma. As a result of being marginalized, disenfranchised, and considered less valuable because of their financial, social, or educational status, they suffer from poverty, racial discrimination, corruption, and violence.

Due to my limited knowledge of the statistics from other cultures, I can only speak about the studies I am aware of in the U.S. and England. However, these are likely reflective of the degree of trauma experienced in other societies.

Motor vehicle accidents are a major cause of trauma in North America. For males they are the most frequent form of trauma and for females the second most frequent. In any given year about 2,500 people die in car crashes in Canada and over 43,000 in the United States. There are also more than two and a half million auto accident related injuries in the U.S.

Violent attack in societies not at war is another scourge, and it is escalating. In a national survey in the United States, more than a third of girls and boys ages ten to sixteen reported being a victim of violence in the form of sexual assault, aggravated assault, or attempted kidnapping. Adults are no less vulnerable to community violence. Well over a third have experienced traumatic events, most of which were the result of serious crimes.

It seems that violence knows no boundaries. In Great Britain, members of the clergy have been advised to remove their clerical collars, except when on official duty, in order to reduce their risk of being attacked. In fact, vicars are attacked more frequently than doctors and even probation officers. One study found that 12% of clergy had suffered some form of violence, while in London nearly half of all vicars reported being attacked in the previous twelve months.

Terrorism has recently moved to the forefront of media attention, though its traumatizing effects have been around for decades. Terrorism is defined as the use of violence against the public to create fear for the purpose of intimidation or coercion. Given this definition, it's evident that many nations have used political terrorism to control their citizens. Wealthy nations have also used economic terrorism against developing nations, while powerful nations have used military terrorism against weaker nations, and radical groups of many faiths have used religious terrorism for domination.

Such terrorist tactics have threatened entire societies. Any of these terrorist activities makes a life unpredictable and unsafe, which often causes a sense of helplessness and hopelessness. In the face of such overwhelming fear and intimidation, people begin to question their fundamental view of the world. Somehow life doesn't seem as meaningful, fair, and safe.

HEART-WRENCHING EFFECTS

The trauma created by natural and human causes is more far-reaching than the immediate deaths or injuries. For instance, the violent vortex of war has a devastating effect on every level of our humanity—our body, our mind, and our spirit.

To illustrate, I had the opportunity to live in Bethlehem, on the West Bank, for three years. During that time, I often traveled back and forth from Bethlehem to Jerusalem. On one such trip, when the border was closed to Palestinians, I happened to arrive at a checkpoint at the same time as a young Palestinian woman. She was carrying a newborn, her first child, trying to take it to the hospital in Jerusalem.

The young mother appeared to be around nineteen years old, about the same age as the soldier who met her at the checkpoint. Her attempts to convince him to allow her to cross the border went from talking to pleading to crying.

Seeing the woman's growing desperation, the soldier was obviously moved. It was clear she was sincere in her attempt to take her child to the hospital. As the conversation grew more intense, I noticed that both the young mother and the equally young soldier began to cry together. It was sad to watch, as the soldier could only deny her entry into Jerusalem even though it was completely against his wishes. I was struck by the pain and anguish that both of these young people endured because of political mandates.

When there is violence, all humanity suffers. How sad we haven't yet learned this simple truth that has been trying to reveal itself to us for generations.

FAR-REACHING CONSEQUENCES

In addition to those who are directly exposed to trauma, millions more experience an indirect impact.

Consider how the entire world witnessed the ineffective evacuation of the city of New Orleans, the slowness of the rescue operation, and the lack of social services in the aftermath of Hurricane Katrina in the United States. Recall our shock when we learned of the scope of the tsunami that battered Southeast Asia. Add to these the many traumatic events we learn about in the course of a single year—massive flooding in Bangladesh, an area the size of Belgium underwater in southern Mexico, devastating floods in China, whole towns cut off by floods in England, earthquakes in Pakistan and Peru, plane crashes in various parts of the world. Such events have an impact on millions of people. Not only those who suffer through such experiences, but journalists, providers of humanitarian services, and even the television audience are traumatized.

Said a consultant who came from Houston to work in the recovery effort in New Orleans, "The most surprising thing to me was that when I went home after the first several months, I was overwhelmed with sadness—it caught me totally by surprise! I only experienced the aftermath of Katrina and, of course, my family and home were never touched."

All along the Gulf Coast we have seen how a disaster of this magnitude incurs considerable loss of people's material and financial resources. As a result, any semblance of an orderly life is severely disturbed. This can place an overwhelming strain on the emotional wellbeing of the individuals involved. Not only can it take years to recover economically, it can be a long time before people simply feel safe again.

VICARIOUS TRAUMA

Have you ever watched horror movies until you scared yourself? If we watch horror on television long enough, we can traumatize ourselves to the point of being terrified by a creaky floorboard or a knock on the door.

Our experience with horror movies demonstrates that we don't actually have to be in a war zone or a region where a natural disaster has occurred in order to experience trauma. Global communication means that more and more of us are alert to the suffering of humanity. No generation before ours has been exposed to such a massive amount of trauma. The death and tragedy we see and hear about in our era is multiple times greater than that of any era before us.

Think back to the falling of the Twin Towers in New York. Each of the towers only fell once, but we all watched them fall over and over on television, generating vicarious trauma. In the end an entire nation was fearful, as though they were the next to be annihilated. People everywhere were suddenly afraid to fly. Discrimination against "Arab-looking" individuals increased dramatically, even though people had never been ill-treated by such people.

Trauma is indelibly imprinted in the psyche of our generation in a way never before possible. Daily exposure to large-scale and long-term experiences of trauma via the media is producing a culture of trauma. This has been described as a "shock to the cultural tissue of a society."[8]

While on the one hand the media provides us with images of destructive events throughout the world so that we are moved to assist those affected by a tragedy, on the other hand awareness of global tragedy is having a deleterious effect on the human psyche. Because images of global crises are so prevalent, we either tune out because we tell ourselves we "can't take anymore," or the threat of terrorism and the like comes to dominate our thoughts.

WEARING US DOWN

Compassion fatigue is a common experience of people who work in trauma-inducing professions, live in violent environments, or are constantly exposed to the needs of suffering people through the media.

This form of fatigue involves an unconscious change in one's own thinking due to exposure to other people's traumatic stories. This phenomenon was first studied among counselors, religious leaders, and medical professionals working in war-torn countries. It was recognized that although a bombing or shooting may have happened just once, professionals often listen to stories of the event numerous times during the week from their clients, patients, or parishioners. This can have a cumulative effect, precipitating fear, anger, or emotional anguish in individuals even though they didn't experience the trauma themselves.

Shootings in public places such as schools, malls, and restaurants are a case in point. Unfortunately these are becoming more common. In a campus shooting, so many students are killed that the families associated with the institution attend funeral after funeral, make numerous hospital visits to either their or their neighbor's children, and visit families and friends to offer consolation. In their attempt to be supportive of others' pain, they often find themselves holding back their own emotions and hiding their tears—as well as trying to control the involuntary shaking that begins when the body is extremely stressed.

After several weeks of this kind of experience, it's natural to feel physically exhausted and emotionally drained. This is because the body contracts the muscles in the face, neck, and torso as a way of holding back tears, thereby controlling our emotions. The best way to lessen this fatigue is to express the emotions that well up at the time of the event or shortly thereafter. Once we allow ourselves to cry and provide the body with sufficient rest, it begins to restore itself.

10

Am I Going Crazy?

❀ ❀ ❀ ❀ ❀

WE DOVE THROUGH THE DOORWAY just before the mortar shell hit the spot where we were sitting seconds earlier. Dirt, mud, and stones splattered our backs. We scrambled frantically on our hands and knees down the short hallway and took cover around the bend in the hallway. Shielding our heads with our hands, sitting in a fetal position, we waited until the shelling stopped some fifteen minutes later.

I would only come to realize two years later that multiple war experiences like these were creating traumatic reactions in me that would in due course manifest as post-traumatic stress disorder.

A PERSONAL EXPERIENCE

When I returned to the United States after having lived in Lebanon for a year during the height of its violence, I began experiencing severe physical and psychological reactions that at first appeared inexplicable.

On one occasion, I went into a department store with my sister-in-law. Someone immediately greeted us with a shopping cart. At the same time, I noticed that the line where you return items for exchange or a refund had a dozen people in it and only one person helping. I was enraged at the injustice of welcoming us to the store and then making us wait to be served.

This simple experience unleashed an inner rage that possessed an uncontrollable intensity. I found myself yelling at my sister-in-law about the injustices of the world. My sister-in-law actually grabbed me by the hands and shouted, "Dave! We're just in a department store!" When I realized the depth of dangerous emotions I had tapped into, I left the store to retreat into the safety and seclusion of my home. I didn't understand my reaction. It made me feel like I was going crazy.

During this time in my life, post-traumatic stress disorder was not well recognized among therapists, so I felt misunderstood and isolated in my quest to discover what was "wrong" with me. Eventually I found a therapist who knew the theory of this disorder but wasn't experienced in any particular methodology to help resolve its symptoms. After several years of inner searching, I unearthed a number of issues that were plaguing me. These issues aren't uncommon in society today, particularly among those who work in trauma-inducing professions such as the military, police, fire fighters, emergency response teams, domestic violence counselors, doctors, nurses, and emergency room personnel.

HOME FROM THE BATTLEFRONT

A soldier's homecoming from war ought to be a joyous event. Yet for many families it's one more traumatic episode.

Returning military personnel can often be distracted by memories of the fighting. Their adrenal responses may still be highly activated, their body tense and contracted. Because the body is energetically charged and prepared for danger, the person is likely to be volatile, defensive, and emotionally distant. Consequently, their reaction to minor stress is exaggerated. After working with over 500 soldiers returning from Iraq and Afghanistan, I recognized that the plane flight home was not long enough to reduce their startled reactions and restore their sense of inner calmness.

This lack of integration time contributed to the increase of domestic violence in families of soldiers who returned from the Gulf War and within a matter of months were being arrested for violent behavior. These otherwise normal, caring men and women who had been role models in the military suddenly found their personalities hijacked by instinctual and uncontrollable chemical reactions in their bodies.

CLUES TO TRAUMA-INDUCED BEHAVIOR

Since trauma-induced behavior tends to embed itself in the person's natural characteristics, an active individual may simply become more active and a quiet individual may become more secluded.

A family member may say to me, "Johnny has always kept to himself. But since the accident, he seems to be a bit more introspective."

The expression "a bit more" is a clue to trauma-induced behavior. I want to know why the individual is "a bit more." If the "bit more" has manifested itself after a traumatic episode, there's a likelihood it's a manifestation of post-traumatic stress disorder.

Only about one out of four who are exposed to trauma develop post-traumatic stress disorder. Why do some fall prey to this and not others?

It's a question of personal history. When you see a person with traumatic symptoms, yet there really is no reason for it, you have to look back at the rest of their life. A traumatic birth, abuse in childhood, multiple surgical procedures or an accident as a child, a divorce early in childhood, mental illness or alcoholism in the family—all of these predispose a person to vulnerability.

It may surprise you that another common symptom of post-traumatic stress disorder is the whiplash associated with automobile accidents. Though the accident may have happened at low speed, and there is really no physical reason for the whiplash, the person is nevertheless in pain. The explanation for this is that whiplash can more likely occur when an individual is vulnerable to trauma because of earlier experiences in their life. In such a vulnerable state, a minor collision at ten miles per hour can cause the person to freeze. If they don't discharge the freeze response, muscle spasm pain occurs. Accident victims who tremor afterwards can more likely discharge the energy and thereby avoid whiplash symptoms.

BREAKING THE SILENCE

Because of ignorance many people suffer in isolated silence, with family and friends wondering, "Why can't they just let it go and move on with their lives?"

For instance, I received an urgent call from the faculty of a school in Africa that had over 200 boys who were war refugees and had been boy soldiers. The students' extreme behavior, involving uncontrollable outbursts of anger, hyperactivity, depression, and absenteeism, were placing a strain on the faculty.

My first step was to gather the entire student body and ask, "How many of you sleep all night long?" Not one student raised his hand. When I asked why they weren't sleeping well, they revealed that they all suffered from chronic nightmares or intrusive memories. Even when the boys were sleeping, if they heard another student in the dormitory having nightmares, they would wake him up and help calm him down. Not one student had slept through an entire night without waking for one disturbing reason or another, yet none of the faculty had any awareness of the endless nights of agony the boys were going through.

After continued questioning of both the students and the faculty, I discovered that the children suffered from other symptoms of post-traumatic stress disorder, such as lack of concentration and short-term memory loss. The faculty were shocked. None of them were aware of the stress these students were enduring.

My first task was to educate the faculty by drawing on their own experiences of vicarious trauma. As the faculty members realized that they themselves were victims of this overwhelming refugee situation, the guilt, anger, and hurt they had experienced was quickly replaced by a sense of renewal, understanding, and self-acceptance.

Once the faculty had been restored to a healthy level of functioning, we redesigned the school's curriculum and class schedule. An important aspect of the redesign was the inclusion in the normal physical education classes of The Trauma Release Process™, which has the ability to release deep chronic tension. This helped the boys discharge the high adrenal and cortisol levels created as a result of their experiences.

We also shortened the teaching segments of each class by introducing five-minute breaks every twenty minutes. This enabled the students to concentrate for the full segment and eventually for the entire class period.

Introducing small study groups allowed the boys to learn at their own pace, which eventually enhanced long-term memory. As the boys struggled in unison to regain their natural cognitive processes, they experienced a sense of cohesion.

Finally, we included a storytelling class in the curriculum. This was specifically designed to elicit the multitude of traumatic memories of these young men in a way that they could feel supported and safe.

These adjustments, over time, reduced and even dismantled many of the neurological, physiological, and psychological defenses these children developed during their time as boy soldiers.

THE WOMEN'S MOVEMENT OPENED OUR EYES

It would be a huge oversight to close this chapter without acknowledging the substantial contribution of the women's liberation movement to our awareness of post-traumatic stress disorder.

With the advent of the women's movement, the traumatic symptoms suffered by women, known previously only as the "problem without a name,"[9] finally received the recognition they deserved. Post-traumatic stress disorder had been studied extensively among soldiers and veterans of war. Only in the 1970s, however, did feminists raise our awareness that the most common traumatic experiences are among women who have suffered domestic violence, rape, and sexual abuse. As a result of women speaking out against the violence they used to endure in silence, a new era of social consciousness dawned.

Awareness of post-traumatic stress disorder among women and children led to recognition of the socialized forms of this affliction that are embedded in the very fabric of society.

II

Resolving Post-Traumatic Stress Disorder

❀ ❀ ❀ ❀ ❀

TRAUMA-INDUCED BEHAVIOR cannot be rectified with the use of traditional crisis intervention techniques that depend on logical processing because trauma behavior is an illogical, instinctual response not under control of the rational brain.

With advances in the field of neurology, science has recognized that this disorder isn't simply about the content of the mind. It's most importantly about how the mind processes that content.

Trauma research has entered a new era that combines the study of the psychology, neurology, and physiology of the individual. This is a refreshing change from the way the mind and body have traditionally been pitted against each other.

OVERWHELMING STRESS

One of the greatest breakthroughs in understanding stress, anxiety, and post-traumatic stress disorder has been in the area of biology.[10] We now know, not merely in theory but through actual measurement, how psychological processes are linked with neurophysiological processes and brain structures.

It turns out that post-traumatic stress disorder symptoms are the result of the same activation of the hypothalamus-pituitary-adrenal axis and the sympathetic or parasympathetic nervous system that occurs during stressful events. In other words, post-traumatic stress symptoms are created by the identical stress hormones released in normal stressful moments.

Post-traumatic stress disorder causes chemical changes in the central nervous system that have a direct biological effect on health. The long-term and cumulative effects of these chemical changes can result in vulnerability to hypertension, immune deficiency, immune disorders, and infections. Additionally, the increase of adrenaline and the decrease of endorphins have a significant effect on muscle tension and how we perceive pain.

The distinguishing feature of post-traumatic stress disorder is that because a situation is believed to be life threatening, our chemical response is much more intense.[11] Whereas our body's response to normal stress can be resolved once the stressful event has ended, post-traumatic stress symptoms tend to persist long after the trauma is over.

"MY BODY IS RACING AT 1000 RPM"

Levels of adrenaline, cortisol, and serotonin are significantly altered when individuals are exposed to prolonged or repeated experiences of trauma.

A soldier described this state: "It's like I'm running at 1000 rpm, and everyone else around me is idling at 30 rpm. I feel all wound up inside and don't have anywhere to discharge this energy." He could not have been more accurate. He was in fact on a chemical high commonly known as an adrenaline rush.

We have all experienced this adrenaline rush. In its wake, we typically calm ourselves down, resume normal life, and see our adrenaline return to its baseline. But when we experience prolonged or repeated stress, this may not happen. Because we continually produce higher levels of adrenaline, our body adjusts to producing these higher levels. After repeated exposure to threatening situations, the body becomes so accustomed to producing high levels of adrenaline and cortisol that it automatically raises the baseline production of these substances. In effect, we become *addicted to our own chemicals.*

Although medical practitioners are well aware of the adrenaline rush created during traumatic experiences, little attention is given to reducing the adrenal and cortisol levels of traumatized individuals. Not only military personnel, but also people living and working in traumatizing environments—such as police, fire fighters, and EMTs—need a way of stabilizing the significant biochemical changes that occur in their bodies as a result of their profession. Victims of domestic violence, such as battered wives and abused children, are other examples of people whose chemistry needs adjustment.

Excess adrenaline production is accompanied by a reduction in serotonin. Serotonin is the "feel good" drug in the body. It's the chemical that inhibits us from acting on our aggressive impulses. A decrease in serotonin in humans has been correlated with impulsivity and aggression. The combination of increased adrenaline and decreased serotonin is precisely what causes an otherwise controlled and calm individual to act out aggressive emotions.

In times of war, danger, or trauma, we need high levels of adrenaline and low levels of cortisol. This combination guarantees we'll have the necessary aggressive feelings to act in our defense. Though such a response keeps us alive in the face of threat, a difficulty arises when we leave the threatening situation and return to a normal environment with our adrenaline and cortisol levels still unbalanced.

THE OPIUM SENSATION

Although we are familiar with the experience of an adrenaline rush, other less-familiar yet significant chemical changes take place in the body during traumatic episodes. The chemicals involved belong to a group known as opioids.

During the attack on the Twin Towers, many who were within proximity of Ground Zero described their experiences in the following ways: "I saw it happening but it was like it wasn't real," "It all seemed to be happening in slow motion," "I ran but I didn't feel like I was in my own body—it was like someone else was running," "I heard screaming but it was surreal," "Although I was badly cut, I didn't feel any pain until it was all over and someone else had to tell me I was hurt."

Such statements in any other circumstance would cause suspicion that the individual was on some kind of mind-altering drug. In fact, this is exactly what's happening. The body has the ability to manufacture mind-and-sensory-altering drugs during a time of trauma.

For example, if we encounter a lion in the jungle and there's no option but to fight it, our adrenaline output shoots up in order to increase muscle tone. However, if our arm is clawed as we fight, our body instantly pumps opioids into the wound so we don't feel the pain. Only after the lion has either been defeated or driven away does the body stop injecting opioids into the arm. We then become aware of the pain, which causes us to seek medical assistance.

Similarly, a soldier on a battlefield may be seriously wounded yet not feel the wound right away. There are many stories of injured combat troops continuing to rush into battle, perhaps to throw a grenade, when they would normally have gone down instantly from the intense pain of such a wound.

Individuals who survive physical abuse often report, "It was as though I was out of my body watching it happen." Or they comment, "I screamed, but it seemed like someone else screaming." Such experiences are opioid-induced.

It's helpful to realize that the body isn't concerned with how we survive trauma, only that we survive. The body will give up and allow itself to be abused if this is the only way it's possible to come through an experience alive. In such a situation, it stops pumping adrenaline—which is causing us to fight, and thereby increasing the degree of danger we are in—and begins pumping opioids so we will collapse, allowing ourselves to be abused but at least live. Thus survivors often report, "I fought and fought, but at some point my muscles gave in and my body simply went limp."

A ONE-TWO PUNCH

In some cases, both adrenaline and opioids work either together or in rapid succession.[12] Such was the case with a Kenyan man who was at the U.S. Embassy in Nairobi when it was bombed. He reacted by going into a state of fight-or-flight coupled with dissociation. He literally ran for a full kilometer without knowing he was running and without knowing where he was going. When people finally stopped him, he sat on the ground and asked, "Where am I?"

The man was bleeding severely from a huge gash in his upper leg. In normal circumstances, this type of injury wouldn't allow a person to walk, let alone run a kilometer. When the gash was pointed out, the man screamed in pain. Until that moment, he hadn't felt the wound. Such is the power of the combination of adrenaline and opioids.

Another common experience among traumatized people is that they swing back and forth from a dissociated or depressed condition to a highly charged state of hyper-arousal. Life is going along fine, until someone makes a slightly critical remark, causing the individual to fly off the handle.

Their rage is accompanied by screaming about "always being picked on." Yet, a short time later, the same individual will again be depressed and despondent even in the face of the most positive comments.

Under the influence of chemical changes, an individual can be social and engaging in the morning but by noon want to isolate themselves. Without knowing the person's trauma history, one could easily suspect some kind of mood disorder. In fact, this condition is often mistaken for manic-depression or bipolar disorder. In a non-clinical sense, it is a bipolar state, because the person swings unpredictably between one pole and the other. But the cause isn't the natural disposition of the individual; it's a post-trauma reaction stemming from an imbalance of chemicals.

WHY WE SOMETIMES FREEZE UP

In the face of an event that causes us to feel helpless, we may freeze up. In such a state, we are unable to draw upon our usual resilience to deal with the threat we are facing. We find ourselves immobilized.

We can see how this works when, in a laboratory, we rub the belly of a frog so it will become motionless, which allows us to study it. The frog is actually going into a freeze. This is a perfectly safe state for a frog, which is capable of hibernating in mud for a whole winter with a heartbeat as low as two or three beats a minute. But for mammals, the freeze is a dangerous state unless it's discharged.

When mammals freeze, the brain releases endorphins that act as anaelgesics—much like taking painkillers. These have the effect of numbing us. In such a condition, the parasympathetic nervous system is dominant, which creates a vegetative state.

It's vital to go through a freeze discharge because it serves as a means of *reliving the trauma in a safe manner.* This way it doesn't become stuck in our memory, where it can be triggered over and over again for years to come. The energy is discharged instead of trapped.

Consider a polar bear that finds itself being followed by a helicopter. Seeing the helicopter as a potential predator, the bear's initial reaction—since it cannot fight the helicopter—is flight. But as the helicopter continues its chase, the bear becomes exhausted, slows down, then collapses onto the ground. It has entered into a freeze.

As the bear comes out of the freeze, it begins to shake violently. Simultaneously, while still lying on its back or side, its paws begin "running" in the air. In other words, the polar bear is doing the thing it was doing when it went into the freeze—only now, it's as if the bear were escaping! By successfully reliving the actions it was going through during its flight, the bear discharges the energy triggered by the trauma.

Unlike polar bears, some animals don't go through a freeze discharge, and this leads to trouble. When an animal doesn't discharge the freeze response, it loses its resilience, lowering its capacity to deal with future threats. Animals that don't discharge the freeze include those in zoos, those in laboratories, domestic animals such as pets and livestock, and humans because we have been socialized not to do so. Each of these animals lives in some form of caged environment—whether a physical cage, or a cultural cage that uses the norms and institutions of society to inhibit them. Consequently, each of these creatures suffers from a variety of physical and psychological complaints.

When we freeze, we may experience an intense sense of unreality, an out-of-body state, clumsiness, amnesia, forgetting who we are, multiple personalities, or a distorted perception of time in which either time seems to stand still or our whole life passes before our eyes in an instant.

The freeze response in mammals can even result in death. The heart relaxes to the point of stoppage. Voodoo death in indigenous tribes has been attributed to this freeze response. Being cursed by a witchdoctor or shaman leads to shunning. Since the social bonding of the tribe is critical to the survival of each member, such shunning can send the person into a freeze, culminating in death.

IDENTIFYING POST-TRAUMATIC STRESS DISORDER

Ongoing post-trauma reactions are caused by the residual undischarged excitement generated at the time of the traumatic event. If the muscles that contracted during the trauma don't release their charge shortly afterwards, they will continue to try to do so at a later date as a way of restoring the body to a restful state.

If this high state of aroused energy is prevented from being discharged, it remains trapped in a bio-neural-physical feedback loop that causes repetitive compulsive behavior. Until the body shakes out this tension, it will continue to repeat this chronic pattern of protection and defense.

Manifestations of this disorder include, but are not limited to, intrusive and recurring recollections of the event, distressing dreams that revolve around the event, efforts to avoid thoughts, feelings, or activities associated with the event, feelings of detachment, a restricted range of feeling, irritability and outbursts of emotion, an exaggerated startle response, hyper-vigilance, and difficulty falling or staying asleep.

12

"Things Like That Don't Happen to Us"

❀ ❀ ❀ ❀ ❀

MORE VIETNAM VETERANS HAVE COMMITTED SUICIDE than soldiers were killed in Vietnam. This is an appalling and shameful statistic.

The rate is so high because, even though post-traumatic stress disorder has been recognized in veterans for decades, the United States doesn't possess a national awareness program or recovery plan to assist soldiers in their reintegration into society. This is unfortunately still the case despite the thousands of soldiers returning from Iraq and Afghanistan who exhibit clear signs of post-traumatic stress disorder.

In the United States, 3.6 days of work impairment per month are associated with post-traumatic stress disorder. This translates into an annual productivity loss in excess of $3 billion.

If one considers all the potentially traumatic events that befall the people of just the American nation in a single year—hurricanes, tornadoes, earthquakes, wildfires, car accidents, sudden deaths, domestic violence, rape, sexual abuse, poverty—it's astounding that the government hasn't instituted a national awareness and recovery plan to assist those individuals affected.

What could possibly be our resistance to offering such a plan to schools, hospitals, emergency services, and national relief agencies?

FLAWED ASSUMPTIONS

In the face of recent large-scale disasters, such as the tsunami in the Indian Ocean, mass flooding and wildfires in many parts of the world, and the Twin Towers and Hurricane Katrina in the United States, there is growing awareness that tragedy can strike anywhere. This is a significant shift in the public's perception, which has tended to see traumatic events as happening to others, elsewhere.

Ingrained deeply in our psyche is a belief that we ourselves are immune to trauma. Behind this belief in our indestructibility is a set of assumptions about the nature of reality. At some level, most of us feel that if we are basically good people, terrible things won't happen to us. We also tend to feel that if a tragedy befalls someone, the person in some way deserved it.

Though these widely held assumptions may seem harmless, they are in fact pernicious. Our private adherence to such illusions not only leaves us completely unprepared to deal with the tragedies of life when they come our way, it is precisely what keeps us from establishing a national system to address trauma. People who see themselves as invincible have no need to establish trauma recovery programs because they are not expecting traumatic experiences to befall them.

Integrity calls us to recognize that trauma can overtake anyone. The Columbine High School tragedy is a case in point. When locals were interviewed shortly after the incident, their comments consisted of statements such as, "We are a quiet middle class neighborhood. Things like this don't happen here." The families associated with the school found themselves ill prepared to deal with the fact that trauma happens to people in every walk of life. The attack shattered the assumption that terrible things don't happen to good people.

People also made statements such as, "Why did this happen to us? We didn't do anything to deserve this." No, the people associated with most traumatic events didn't do anything to deserve such terrible tragedies. This statement of disbelief contradicts society's widely held assumption that people get what they deserve in life. Those close to the victims found it no longer possible to comfort themselves with the idea that bad things only happen to others.

Since many of our religious beliefs are based on the premise that people deserve what they get, and that bad things only happen to bad people, many loose faith in their religion and their God when trauma forces its way into their lives.

The kind of "peace of mind" that results from living in an illusion is easily shattered. Far better to search within ourselves and face up to our hidden fear of our precarious position on this planet. Then, we can *learn to live with unpredictability* rather than fantasizing that if we just "do the right thing," we can somehow prevent trauma from entering our lives. As long as we don't come face to face with life's unpredictability, we will likely avoid instituting a national trauma awareness program and plans to assist those traumatized members of society in need of help.

Until we recognize that the social cost of post-traumatic stress disorder outweighs the financial cost of healing our citizens, we will continue to deny the need for large-scale trauma recovery programs.

TRAUMATIZED CHILDREN BECOME TRAUMATIZED ADULTS

If, as a society, we respond to adult trauma inadequately, our response to trauma in the lives of children is even more woeful.

Commented one researcher, "It is an ultimate irony that at the time when the human is most vulnerable to the effects of trauma—during infancy and childhood—adults generally presume the most resilience."[13]

This destructive misperception that children are more resilient than adults has permeated the mental health field for years. For example, even though our response to adult trauma has been inadequate, during the last decade we have spent billions of dollars studying and treating adult trauma victims, primarily male combat veterans, while few resources have been dedicated to research or treatment focused on childhood trauma—even though millions of children around the world are continually exposed to traumatic experiences.

It's estimated that more than a million and a half children per year are maltreated. Conservative estimates of the number of children in the United States exposed to a traumatic event in a single year exceed four million. These include children who live in the fallout zone of domestic or community violence, have experienced physical or sexual abuse, have witnessed or experienced violent crime, or have been exposed to other unexpected violence such as car accidents, burn accidents, kidnappings, or other forms of attack.

At least half of all children exposed to traumatic experiences develop a variety of significant symptoms in adolescence and adulthood. Depending on the severity, frequency, and nature of the trauma, these children are at risk for developing serious emotional, physical, cognitive, and behavioral problems.

When children experience trauma while the brain is in its developmental stages, they devise coping strategies to help them get through the trauma. Adults do this too. We all come up with ways of dealing with what we are faced with. We will dissociate into fantasy worlds, isolate ourselves from friends, or become overly engaged socially to avoid being alone.

The difference between a mature adult in a healthy mental state and a developing child is that the adult has the ability to dismiss the coping strategy once it has served its purpose. To an otherwise developed brain, this coping strategy functions as a band-aid. But the developing brain in a child cannot distinguish between a coping strategy, which serves a temporary purpose, and a pattern of behavior that becomes built into the brain as a permanent characteristic.

If children grow up in a traumatic environment, the more they are forced to use patterns of thought that help them cope with trauma. It's also more likely that those patterns will become embedded in their natural thought processes and become lifelong traits.

Traumatized children then begin to process all unfamiliar and overwhelming events as though these events had the potential of being dangerously traumatizing. This causes them to overact to normal events, producing hyper-arousal and even what clinicians call "dissociative behavior." This is when children develop secret places in their minds where they go when overwhelmed. Such places are often highly fanciful, bearing little resemblance to reality. In terms of the real world, the child has shut down. The result is often a vacant stare, curling up in a fetal position, or rhythmic rocking, stroking, or bumping.

School teachers, administrators, and other personnel within the educational system are left to deal not only with the maladaptive behavior of the traumatized children they teach, but also with the vicarious trauma they themselves develop as a result of being exposed to the children's symptoms on a daily basis.

Given these daunting statistics, educators and school personnel should at least be provided with the opportunity to educate themselves on the symptoms and effects of trauma, as well as to learn preventive protocols. But it is also essential that society tackle the roots of the problem.

REVERSING GENERATIONS OF NEGLECT

All societies have neighborhoods that are particularly susceptible to the development of stress, anxiety, and trauma. Such neighborhoods are usually populated by people who have been marginalized by political oppression, poverty, discrimination, or poor education.

Marginalized environments often become fallout zones for domestic or community violence. Individuals who have been disenfranchised by the dominant culture of a society find themselves trapped in ghettos of human degradation.

The heightened trauma induced by such environments tends to become a unifying force, binding marginalized groups of society into tight communities, so that few ever find a route of escape. Grinding poverty and violence become hallmarks of daily existence.

How can society ever reverse generations of neglect, given the entrenched disdain for human worth with which such environments are riddled?

Couple this with the unwillingness of most of us even to think about what might be needed to change such a situation—as long as it does not spill over into more affluent neighborhoods.

A UNIQUE BAND OF PEOPLE

There exists within society a band of people who, since the inception of their profession, have traditionally crossed the boundaries between diverse populations, seeking to bring healing where others fear to tread. We call them social workers.

Since its foundation by Mary Richmond and Jane Addams, social work has had its roots embedded in the locales where stress, anxiety, and trauma most adversely affect both the individual and society. Whether in settlement houses or in ethnic neighborhoods, social workers have often lived and worked in environments where life is challenging.

While traditional counseling generally addresses only the psychological and emotional elements of stress, social workers have an awareness and concern for the biological and social state of their clients as well as their psychological condition. But despite the growing awareness of the connection between an individual's biological, psychological, and sociological wellbeing, bodily intervention still tends to fall outside the domain of social work. Even though many physical maladies are reported by people experiencing a variety of stressful and anxiety-producing events, social workers are often hesitant to recommend body-oriented interventions.

It's precisely because the social work profession continually crosses the boundaries of diverse populations that social workers have the potential to bring integrated solutions to the burgeoning problems of stress, anxiety, and trauma. In our era of escalating trauma, it's important that social workers possess a working knowledge of body-based interventions. By utilizing bodywork in conjunction with counseling, the social worker's effectiveness is enhanced. Treatment is not only more effective but also reduced in duration. When social workers are aware of body-based interventions such as Trauma Release Process™ techniques, they are well positioned to bring a much-needed body-based intervention to the attention of their clients.

A PRICE WE CAN AFFORD

Due to the increase in psychologically based mental health disorders in the United States even in otherwise healthy individuals, there is great interest on the part of the medical community and the government in more cost-effective, self-directed therapies. For instance, we have already seen that there is heightened interest in exercise as an alternative or adjunct to traditional interventions such as psychotherapy or drug therapies.

Because the method I put forth in this book is easy to teach and learn, it can be used as a self-directed exercise routine. Since there is no need for special materials or therapeutic supervision, the method is cost-effective and therefore available even to large populations within the lower socio-economic bracket.

This approach also has implications for self-directed stress reduction exercises for many professionals who work in stress-inducing professions. Many of these individuals don't presently seek counseling for fear that it could harm their career, cause them to have difficulties with their peers or superiors, or be a stigmatizing admission of an inherent weakness of character. A self-directed, body-based method of stress reduction allows individuals to process their own stress without needing to seek the guidance of professionals.

The time has never been as ripe for the government to institute a national plan for trauma awareness and recovery, utilizing the skilled individuals who are already present where they are most needed. All that is needed is the will to provide the necessary additional training and monitoring for such a program.

At every level, a national strategy is demanded—for schools, for people in trauma-inducing professions, for returning military personnel, and for all who suffer post-traumatic stress disorder. It's in our best interest to provide such assistance because not only are traumatized individuals a potential danger to themselves and to others, but trauma behavior and symptoms can be passed on to our children—a phenomenon that is increasing in society at an alarming rate and for which we are all paying a high price.

As we become a global community, there are signs that some nations are beginning to grapple with and support one another in their attempts to deal with and heal local, national, and international experiences of trauma.

It's all the more crucial that we address this situation, given that today we at last have an understanding of how post-traumatic stress disorder is triggered—and what to do about it when it occurs.

13

Trauma in the Workplace

❁ ❁ ❁ ❁ ❁

CORPORATIONS AND OTHER LARGE ORGANIZATIONS that employ people are primed to begin establishing large-scale plans for trauma recovery because they have much to lose if they don't and the potential of much to gain if they do.

The effects of post-traumatic stress disorder in the workplace can be so severe that it's economically imperative to treat this condition. Unless trauma is resolved, it can mercilessly fracture the cohesion of even the best-led teams and corporate relationships.

TRUST IS ESSENTIAL

If we belong to a social club, a religious institution, or a political group, the ability to function effectively together for the common good is grounded in trust. When we can't trust the club president, our minister or rabbi, or the leader of a political group, it's difficult to get much done. The discord that results often drives good group members away.

If we glance at profiles on singles' dating sites, one of the elements of character people seek most in a partner is someone they can trust. We want to know that the person we are partnered with romantically will be honest with us, straightforward, aboveboard, and transparent. "No games, no lies!"

The same is true of people we are partnered with in business. If we are to entrust our financial wellbeing to them, we need to know we can count on them.

In our modern economy, it's crucial to be able to function effectively as a member of a team. When people can't pull together as a team, they undermine the endeavor in which they are engaged. In *The Five Dysfunctions of a Team,* teamwork expert Patrick Lencionis identifies lack of trust as the first obstacle to effective teamwork. Whether you work in an office, a factory, or in the service industry, trust is essential in the workplace.

ENCODED NOT TO TRUST

When people break trust, it's difficult to restore a relationship. There's been a qualitative shift that forever generates doubt, no matter how much the untrustworthy individual seeks to reassure us. We want to trust them again, but something in our gut remains guarded. The distrust doesn't easily go away.

Even the most clever strategies, insightful crisis management techniques, and sharpest of business acumen can prove unable to rectify the damage individuals do to each other once trauma infects the corporate domain.

Lack of trust is such a difficult barrier to overcome that many organizations engage in a variety of mental exercises to try to restore trust among their employees. This is often of only limited success because traumatized individuals have a neural impediment to trusting that's tainted with a life-or-death prospect. They are neurologically encoded *not* to trust, for fear that their openness will expose them to a similar life-or-death situation. Since this is unconscious and many people are unaware of this psychic mandate, they cannot trust even when they actually prefer to do so.

This is where the Trauma Release Process™ can play a helpful role.

For instance, I was asked to go to Sudan to work with a Muslim and Christian population in the city of Khartoum. The invitation was from a nonprofit organization. I was to work with two people who were co-leaders in the organization.

I began by hearing about the animosity between the two individuals, which was typically reflective of the culture. "We are experiencing division that we believe is coming from our culture and not from us individually," said one of the participants. "Even though we want to move beyond these divisions, our animosity is so deeply entrenched that we don't seem to be able to pull ourselves out of it."

"If it's coming from the culture," I explained, "then you need to have a shared experience that restores your commonality as human beings."

I offered to lead them through such an experience, and they agreed to participate.

"How, in your bodies, do you know that you are experiencing animosity?" I asked. "What, exactly, does it feel like?"

"I feel that my chest is tight, and I don't breathe deeply because I'm not relaxed," said one of the participants. "My shoulders are tight, my neck is tense, and I sense I have a lot of anxiety in my body that I can't release."

The other was shocked to hear what his fellow worker was experiencing. "That's exactly how I feel!" he exclaimed.

"You are having a common experience because all humans feel separation and division by means of an identical bodily process,"

I explained. "What you are both doing is separating yourselves from your bodies. The way to change this is for both of you to have an identical bodily experience that's positive."

At this point I invited them to do the Trauma Release Process™ I developed. I positioned them so they could both see each other doing the exercises. When they both began to tremor part way into the exercises, they realized that their bodies were responding in the same manner.

"What's going on in your body right now?" I asked.

The first man said, "I can feel my legs are tremoring from my feet up to my hips."

"Wow!" said the second man. "That's exactly what's happening to me."

This second man then described a different sensation. "I find myself tremoring in my stomach," he said. "At the same time, I'm also beginning to feel my breath deepening."

"The identical sensation is happening in me," said the second man.

"Yes, our bodies are responding in exactly the same way," agreed the other.

These two men were actually mirroring each other. I kept them tremoring against the wall for quite a while so they could experience how their bodies were acting in concert with each other.

"Your bodies are discharging the identical tension you were experiencing in your work together," I explained.

"My God," they both exclaimed, "we are so alike!"

Once I was able to get them to see that they were alike, it dismantled their conceptualization that they were so different. The animosity was now no longer there because they recognized they were essentially very similar to one another.

Once they restored a sense of their commonality, I had them lie on the floor for a final exercise. The tremors that arose from this exercise evoked laughter in both men, to the point that they ended up with deep belly laughs. When they at last stood, they hugged each other, aware that they no longer had any sensation of animosity in their bodies.

There was nothing to work through, no deep analysis required. They simply needed to discharge what had been put onto them by their culture.

SIGNS OF TRAUMA IN THE WORKPLACE

The second of the five dysfunctions of a team identified by Lencionis is fear of conflict. Fear is natural, and in the normal course of things it can be overcome through skilled management techniques. But in the case of traumatized individuals, overcoming fear isn't so easy.

A traumatized individual tends to lack the ability to rate their fears on a graded scale and thereby put them in perspective. When a person lacks the normal gradations of feeling, *any* occurrence of fear is immediately translated into terror. The individual's reaction will be overly defensive, likely in the form of an outburst of anger, tears, or withdrawal into isolation and even depression.

The Five Dysfunctions of a Team identifies the other three dysfunctions as lack of commitment, avoidance of accountability, and inattention to results. Each of these is an inevitable consequence of being traumatized.

It's vital to be sensitive to the signs of trauma in team members. Such signs are an excessive need to control, becoming less caring about the company's concerns, compulsive perfectionist behavior, and isolating oneself from other employees.

MENDING STRAINED RELATIONSHIPS

I was invited to work with the staff of one of the consulates in Jerusalem. They have a multicultural staff consisting of Muslims, Christians, and Jews. The external tension of the political situation was fragmenting the relationships of their otherwise cohesive team.

The consulate had already tried traditional programs of crisis management, cross-cultural leadership, and conflict resolution in an attempt to heal the strained relationships. All of these failed to rectify the intense divisions that were seriously fracturing their leadership team.

Since it was apparent that each of the staff members had experienced trauma either directly or vicariously, I knew the techniques they had been using would be ineffective. Such techniques fail to take into account the unique characteristics of trauma-induced behavior.

It's not commonly recognized that *trauma-induced behavior is designed to protect traumatized people from additional trauma.* This is why it's so difficult to get traumatized individuals to let go of such behavior.

Because the actions and reactions of trauma victims are mostly instinctual rather than conscious and calculated, reprocessing of the trauma cannot generally be approached in a systematic, logical manner. Attempting conscious and logical resolution of a crisis created by unconscious and illogical reactions renders traditional crisis management ineffective.

The most damaging effect of post-traumatic stress disorder on the consulate staff was the breakdown of trust in their professional relationships. There were increased signs of isolation, and a sense of helplessness and hopelessness—to the point that team members found themselves losing both their concern for each other and their ability to act in a caring way. All of this has devastating effects within and between organizations and corporations.

FOSTERING CORPORATE LONGEVITY

As the CEO of Trauma Recovery Assessment and Prevention Services, I have worked fifteen years with corporate, embassy, government, and non-government personnel who live and serve in trauma-inducing environments. I have observed that trauma and its consequences affect all institutions that have personnel living or working in life-threatening environments. I have also noticed that everyone who experiences trauma suffers from one or more symptoms of post-traumatic stress disorder. It's a prevalent and debilitating condition that doesn't discriminate, and the only difference from one person to another is the degree of suffering.

The need for new trauma resolution options has tremendous implications for corporations and organizations whose personnel are living or working in crisis environments. Only now are we recognizing the long-term, damaging effects trauma has on the fabric of corporations and organizations. Human relations and public relations personnel are finding they are unprepared, ill equipped, and lack the knowledge to adequately address the multifaceted dimensions of this rather severe and large-scale phenomenon.

As a case in point, after 9/11 I asked a number of personnel whose companies were directly affected by this event what type of debriefing and support they had received from their company. Although many were grateful for the support they had been given, they felt it was woefully inadequate. After the initial debriefing, they were told that if they had any additional problems, they should seek out private therapeutic help.

By telling staff to go elsewhere for help, the organization is taking a hands-off approach that sends the message, "Your problem isn't our concern." This has an isolating effect on members of the workforce, causing them to feel as if the organization doesn't care about them. In return, the workforce begins to experience a lack of commitment to the organization. Instead of the trauma drawing team members together, it ends up splintering them into their own isolated worlds. However, when a team works through trauma together, their confidence in their ability to resolve issues rises, which bolsters their sense of competence. In turn, the increased feeling of competence reflects in the team's performance.

Organizations seriously hurt themselves when they treat employees in an uncaring manner. When an employee is treated poorly, the entire workforce takes note. For instance, as an employee, you work loyally for a company, buy a house and car based on your income, then one morning arrive at work to find your job has been eliminated due to downsizing. You can't get into your office because it has been locked. Your personal belongings are in a box. You are told you have two hours to leave and will not be allowed back. You are severed from the people you have worked with, whose response is fear because they all realize that what is happening to you, a friend they care about, could just as easily happen to them.

Of course, a consultant is there to do the dirty work, and relocation counselors are provided to advise you. It's a traumatizing experience—and, shamefully, standard workplace practice. Then corporations expect their remaining employees to pick up and carry on as usual.

To overlook or misunderstand this fundamental issue of large-scale traumatization is to trivialize the emotional complexities facing many international corporations. If left untreated, the long-term effects of unresolved symptoms give rise to forms of dysfunctional behavior that can seriously undermine any team, organization, or corporation.

As anxiety, depression, and anger increase in our world, companies need to be proactive in not only offering their employees education about trauma, but also providing them with effective techniques to assess themselves and resolve their own trauma as it arises.[14]

Due to the unconscious and insidiously eroding effects that trauma has on interpersonal relationships, the corporations that will have the most enduring relationships in the future are those that recognize, respect, and resolve the traumatized behavior and relationships of their personnel. Any corporation that doesn't recognize and respect the devastating potential of trauma on its personnel will not be able to sustain long-term trust.

14

Healing Our Division

❀ ❀ ❀ ❀ ❀

IF RELATIONSHIPS IN CORPORATE AND GOVERNMENT SETTINGS can be seriously disrupted by trauma, it's little wonder that nations have difficulty relating.

Oftentimes the need for international conflict resolution results from the inability of two groups to reconcile with each other because of long-standing wars, political violence, or sectarian armed conflict. Witness the ongoing tension between Turks and Armenians, Palestinians and Israelis, Kurds and Iraqis, Muslims and Christians over conflicts that erupted decades ago.

Since all serious conflict produces years of trauma, most if not all of the participants in a conflict resolution process will have experienced some form of trauma, either directly or vicariously. Participants are likely to bring with them a multitude of unconscious post-traumatic stress behaviors that undermine the reconciliatory process.

RECONNECTING ALIENATED PARTIES

Let me illustrate this from a workshop I conducted with Palestinians and Israelis. The group divided into pairs, first as two Palestinians together and two Israelis together. They were given a series of questions and tasks to work though, which all did with great ease.

The group then divided into pairs of one Palestinian and one Israeli. As they tried to work through the same questions and tasks, they realized it was excruciatingly difficult. The words and phrases they had used with someone from their own ethnic background were no longer safe to use in the mixed group. A simple exercise of setting boundaries with one another erupted in an argument in which intense emotions were expressed. The two parties, although desirous of healthy dialogue, discovered that even their best intentions couldn't override the divisive effect of their thinking, which had been tainted by trauma.

The group was then put through the Trauma Release Process™ and led in a workshop on trauma-induced behavior. As a result of the physical exercises and gaining an understanding of trauma, these two groups were able, with surprising ease, to feel connected, safe, and even emotionally caring towards each other's pain.

The change was astounding. In fact, the two groups could not believe how much they were able to change their thinking, feelings, and behavior by addressing the issue of trauma recovery prior to attempting dialogue and resolution of their conflicts.[15]

"I HATED EVERYONE TO THE POINT OF PARANOIA"

In the late 70s and early 80s, I lived in East Beirut, Lebanon, which was predominantly Christian. I saw firsthand the damage inflicted on us by those living on the west side of Beirut, who were predominately Muslim.

Though I had always sought to be unprejudiced toward different peoples, I found myself developing first an anger toward, and eventually a hatred for, "those Muslims." I knew it was wrong to feel this way, and I fought it. But as the destruction continued, the situation inevitably got the better of me and I became as prejudiced as everyone else.

Then my house was bombed and I was forced to move to the west side of the city where I rented from a wonderful Muslim family with whom I became close friends. Now I was subjected to bombing and shelling from the Christians, and I was witnessing the suffering of Muslims just as I had witnessed the suffering of Christians in my former house. Quite involuntarily, my allegiance began to switch. The hatred I had felt toward Muslims was now projected onto the Christians. They were the new enemy.

I had a similar experience when I encountered conflicts between Palestinians and Israelis, Northern and Southern Sudanese, and Eritreans and Ethiopians. I wondered at how my mind could so readily transfer my allegiance from one group to another. The reality is that discrimination attaches itself to whatever group we feel threatened by at the time.

You can see from my personal experience how easy it is for the different sides in a conflict to become locked into their position. Once violence flares, entrenched animosity is inevitable.

At the same time, my experience in Lebanon contains the seeds of hope. If we can once begin to see from the other's viewpoint, we realize how easily we become polarized. Recognizing this opens a portal for ending the conflict.

HOW WE LEARN TO DISCRIMINATE

Discrimination is an instinctual, protective behavior. All animal species possess this instinct as a means of preserving their species.

It works like this. In more primitive times, when we came across a lion, we learned that this was a potentially life-threatening creature. In order for us not to have to learn this lesson through repeated experiences, the mind applied a discriminating fear to all animals of a similar nature—tigers, panthers, cougars, and jaguars. In this way we learned to discriminate between whole categories of harmful and non-harmful cats. As a primitive species living with the dangers of the jungle, this was a valuable protective mechanism that helped keep our species alive.

This discriminating mechanism continues to be available to us when we are in danger. For instance, it's protective of soldiers when they must instantly identify the "enemy" so that they themselves are not killed.

The trouble is, this mechanism can also be unleashed in everyday life in a manner that backfires. In civilization, the majority of us are no longer endangered by wild animals or on the battlefield. Under normal circumstances, we use the logic of our neocortex to help us make decisions. But when we are threatened in some way, all of us experience activation of this primal mechanism. Our logic gets hijacked by the reptilian brain—the limbic system—which reacts instinctively. This is how much conflict comes about.

STEREOTYPING IS A DEFENSE

When we lose perspective under the impact of a hijacking by the reptilian brain, we resort to stereotyping.

Take the case of a female client recovering from sexual assault who came to my office and announced, "No man can be trusted. I hate all men!"

This is an understandable reaction to having just had one's life threatened by a male. The brain is simply applying its natural protective instinct to anyone who resembles the attacker. As the client progressed in her recovery, her belief that "all" males are dangerous yielded to the logic of her neocortex. She learned to identify some males as potentially dangerous and others as safe.

When the logic and reason of the neocortext doesn't kick in during times of safety, the mechanism of the reptilian brain that gives us a tremendous survival advantage in the face of real danger becomes a liability. For instance, if the reptilian brain has not been quieted, a person from a particular ethnic group who is no threat at all to our physical wellbeing suddenly becomes a threat to our *ego*.

Whatever category of people we feel threatened by will cause the development of an "enemy image" in the mind. This image is then indiscriminately applied to all who appear to fit the image. It expresses itself as fear of black men, fear of Hispanics, fear of homosexuals, fear of women, fear of men, and the like. A whole race can become victims of ethnic cleansing, or a particular nationality become "undesirables," fit only for banning, controlling, humiliating, or even killing.

The current atmosphere of anti-Arab and Muslim sentiment in the United States is a perfect example. Many Americans have taken Arabs and Muslims in general and assumed they are all potential terrorists— and so we discriminate under the guise of "protecting the nation." What's happening is that the more primitive part of our brain is at work in a manner that's no longer appropriate in a sophisticated society.

How ironic that a mechanism that once helped protect the human species and cultivated its survival is now actually dividing and can potentially destroy our species.

With the increasingly multiracial, ethnically diverse, and religiously pluralistic nature of the modern world, it's becoming more crucial that we allow our reptilian brain to relax a little, in order to make way for an expanded self-identity that can be more inclusive of all people.

Along this line, we should remember that not long ago the French were castigated by many Americans for not supporting the attack on Iraq. French fries were renamed "freedom fries," and bottles of French champagne were poured down the drain as Americans projected the French government's stand on a single issue onto the entire nation and citizens of France.

By the same token, France's next president, Nicolas Sarkozy, declared his desire to "reconquer the heart of America" as he was welcomed with open arms on a state visit to Washington. The British *Daily Telegraph* commented that even by the standards of Washington's lavish hospitality, the welcome afforded the French president "has been extraordinary."

When trauma dissipates, we return to our right mind. Our cerebral cortex kicks in, allowing us to use our head instead of losing it. We become truly *discriminating,* and therefore no longer *discriminate* against those whom we have until now seen as somehow subhuman. External conflict comes to a close with the dawn of internal peace.

15

"God No Longer Existed for Me"

❁ ❁ ❁ ❁ ❁

A DEVOTED CHRISTIAN WOMAN WHOSE DAUGHTER had been shot dead came to me shortly after the murder. She told me it was important that she not give up her faith in God as a result of this tragedy. "I'm going to hold onto my belief that Jesus is Lord," she asserted, "and that God had a reason for this to happen."

From having worked with so many people, I knew that this woman was going to have a difficult time holding onto her belief. To try to fit this senseless slaying into her existing faith, without allowing her daughter's tragic end to affect her worldview, was sheer avoidance.

People who try to force trauma into an already established set of beliefs inevitably become rigid in their faith. They try to pray harder, be better, and follow the "rules" more ardently.

In my experience this never works. Unhealed trauma either masks a bitter, angry, resentful individual whose suppressed rage expresses itself through unbending doctrines and harsh practices, or it causes the individual to slide into an apathetic view of all spirituality and abandon the idea of a meaningful faith entirely.

It is only when we engage in the trauma recovery process wholeheartedly that we can rewrite our belief system in a way that our faith is not only restored but deepened and purified by the traumatic event that threw us into our initial doubt and despair.

A SHATTERING EXPERIENCE

We imagine that our worldview—our faith—will stay intact through anything life throws at us. But trauma is something that, until it befalls us, is outside our range of comprehension.

Trauma is an overwhelming and seemingly unbearable experience, and once it enters our life, our understanding of ourselves, our friends and family, and our place in the universe are often drastically altered. In fact, our entire view of life can be forever changed.

The sad reality is that many who go through traumatic events experience a deadening of their spirituality. Their faith is shattered, and they find themselves unable to rebuild it. As one person told me in the wake of a tragedy, "God no longer exists for me."

It doesn't matter whether we are theistic, atheistic, or agnostic, trauma causes us to question. We wonder about our place in the universe in the face of the seemingly capricious and precarious workings of nature.

A SPIRITUAL AWAKENING

While some lose their faith when overwhelming trauma assails, others experience a spiritual transformation. They find themselves not merely reestablishing a damaged faith, but undergoing a profound reorientation of their lives.

In fact, many refer to this deepening of their spirituality as an *awakening*.

"I do not wish tragedy on anyone," said one trauma survivor, "but ever since that accident, I never fail to tell my wife I love her. I kiss my children every day. Life is richer, fuller, and deeper than I have ever experienced. It has more meaning and depth than it ever had before." This type of transformation after surviving a traumatic experience is common.

How does such a painful experience enable us to live a more profound life than we previously did? Why don't we simply choose to live life at its deepest level without having to endure a tragedy? Why do we need to undergo a traumatic experience before we wake up and appreciate life to its fullest?

The questioning process that follows a traumatic time in our lives isn't simply a matter of one's "faith being tested." It's far more complex. When a traumatic experience befalls us, our usual understanding and logic is undermined, and often thrown into serious doubt, under the weight of the trauma. But it's precisely at this point that a natural neurological process kicks in, stimulating the reflective part of the brain— the neocortex—to help us reevaluate our faith.

Anyone who has struggled to recover from a traumatic event knows that they process the event over and over, focusing intensely on the trauma, trying to find some sense in the apparent senselessness. Because the traumatic experience is outside our present worldview and ability to process logically, it seems completely overwhelming and unbearable.

However, it is precisely because it seems overwhelming that we can be forced out of an old way of thinking and eventually into a new way of being in our lives. This process of forced expansion occasions the evolution of our mind. It is this process that invites us to expand our worldview, and in fact demands of us that we do so *in such a manner as to include the traumatic experience*. Such an expanded vision helps us to accept the trauma and incorporate its impact into our life's experiences.

In other words, built right into our human developmental process is the ability to experience trauma and restructure our thinking to embrace the event, make sense of it, and gradually engage life more deeply in the context of a richer and more meaningful worldview.

I have found that even people who don't espouse any particular faith invariably possess some understanding, no matter how vague or undefined, of how they and their life fit into the broader scheme of things.

OUR SPIRITUAL SELF

After having worked with so many survivors from so many different types of trauma, I began recognizing patterns that involved people's belief systems—or what they often referred to as their "faith" or "spirituality." I was curious about these patterns and began asking survivors about any changes they had experienced in their faith.

The most succinct and profound response came from a Catholic nun in Ethiopia. After a workshop I was leading in Addis Ababa, she came to talk with me privately. "Since my experiences with war," she said, "I have not been able to pray, and I am worried about this."

Curious about her statement I asked, "How do you know you can't pray since the war?"

What followed was an amazing insight into the spiritual state of a trauma survivor. "Before the war," she related, "I used to go into the chapel and pray the rosary. I attended mass. I prayed the breviary four times a day. I spoke a lot with God." In short, this woman had performed all the rites and rituals expected of her as a Catholic nun.

"How is your prayer life different now?" I asked.

"Now when I go into the chapel, I simply turn off all the lights and sit in silence," she explained. "I don't have any words. I don't talk to God, and I don't listen to God. I just sit. I don't know what else to do. There don't seem to be any words or thoughts to express my innermost feelings. I don't feel alone or abandoned, I simply sit there."

This nun had expressed in the simplest of terms what so many trauma survivors experience—that there are no words to describe the depth of human experience the trauma survivor has been plunged into. Without knowing how or why, this nun found herself in a realm so few dare to explore. Even though she couldn't make sense of this peculiar place, it was neither frightening nor disconcerting to her. She simply didn't understand it.

"How does it feel to be in this place?" I asked.

"I don't mind it," she said. "It's actually quite peaceful. There is no movement, no action, and no words. I just sit there. I neither feel God's presence nor the absence of God's presence. It isn't particularly spiritual. It just is."

In the wake of her traumatic experience, this sincere human being had been drawn into a place within herself that required a deeper exploration of "self." It is a place of the unknown, and yet the person usually knows they need to be there. I believe it to be a place the person instinctually knows they need to explore in order to develop a greater sense of inner peace. It reminds me of a profound insight I found in a book entitled *Being Peace* by the Buddhist monk Thich Nhat Hanh: "Without being peace, we cannot do anything for peace." Without knowing it, this nun had been drawn into a place where she was exploring inner peace. She was realizing that if she couldn't be peaceful inside, she would not be able to contribute to peace in the world around her.

I have found this same intense need for self-exploration in thousands of people from many countries, cultures, and religious and spiritual backgrounds. After a trauma, even survivors who are self-proclaimed atheists or agnostics seem to go through an inner questioning of their sense of self, their relationship to others, and their relationship to life. It seems to me that this questioning is an innate process and part of our evolutionary journey.

SOLITUDE——A KEY TO REINVENTING OURSELVES

For survivors to engage the process of discovering a deeper identity for themselves after a trauma, I have learned that the presence of a guide can be a lifesaver.

At one point in my own journey when I was recovering from severe post-traumatic stress disorder, I felt a compelling, almost incessant need to escape from the world. I didn't know what this meant or why I needed it. I only knew I had to be in solitude and silence. I didn't want to be around anyone, and I didn't want to talk or listen to anyone.

Because of this unrelenting urge, I found a hermitage in California that granted me permission to live with the monks for six months. When I arrived at the hermitage, the abbot said: "We have a policy here that you cannot live alone in intense silence and solitude without some guidance." I reluctantly agreed to the guidance, not knowing what this would mean. I only came to understand later how helpful external guidance can be.

From the first day I entered the monastery, I lived half of my day in complete silence and solitude, then spent the other half in community service working alongside the other monks in silence. This rhythm was amazingly therapeutic for me. I could feel something inside of me being resolved.

Though I was healing, I didn't know from what, let alone why or how. I simply knew I was becoming more peaceful.

It actually took a full three months of living in this style to realize how noisy and chaotic my thoughts were. My head was buzzing with inner chaos. I was also filled with emotions that were just as chaotic. I went from anger to rage, to sadness, to hatred, to loneliness, to despair, and back again to rage. There seemed to be no rhyme or reason to these emotions. They didn't seem to be attached to anyone or anything in particular. Whether they were toward God, the universe, everyone in my personal life, humanity in general, I honestly didn't know. All I knew was that I felt crazy inside my head and body. Uncontrollable thoughts and emotions overwhelmed me. At times I found myself sitting alone swearing, yelling, enraged, and I didn't know why. I felt officially insane.

At this point I was grateful to have a guide. Had I not had someone to keep me in touch with reality, I would probably have been so carried away by my emotions that I would have committed suicide. These thoughts and emotions were so overwhelming and uncontrollable, they were kidnapping my sanity.

Six months later I left the hermitage. Although my thoughts and emotions still had some elements of uncontrollability, I had a greater sense of peace. My thoughts were not being hijacked as easily and my emotions were not as volatile. I was able to separate my sane moments from my insane moments. What a relief this was. I actually felt I was emerging from some deep inner quagmire of chaos.

This experience was priceless for my recovery from post-traumatic stress. I learned that at some point in my recovery, simply *being* with myself in solitude and stillness was both inevitable and invaluable. I needed to explore "me." No one could do this for me. I had to go inside and see who I really was in light of all I had experienced and done in my life. I was coming to know, or re-know, myself at a deeper level.

I have worked with many trauma survivors in my career as a therapist. This experience has taught me that, at a certain point in the recovery process, each person goes through a phase that requires some kind of reinventing of themselves.

The difficult part of this process is that only we can explore this inner place of pain, anguish, and craziness. We must go there alone. However, it's important to be tethered to a lifeline held by a close friend, therapist, or guide. Going into this place without an objective observer can cause us to get lost in the internal chaos. Having someone who holds the other end of the line of reality facilitates our return to the realm of sanity.

FORGIVING LIFE FOR ITS "FAILINGS"

An important aspect of reinventing ourselves in the wake of trauma, so that we can go on with our lives in an enriched mode, is being able to let go of the past. This requires the ability to forgive.

Trauma release is an act of forgiveness. It may involve forgiving another person, another country, or even Mother Nature herself.

Refusal to forgive leads us into an excruciating double bind. As one researcher put it, "Our refusal to forgive the past imprisons us in our own resistance to our natural, evolutionary instincts and thereby has the power to deny us a healthy movement into our future."[16]

When we forgive instead of blaming, we experience a letting go. This allows for the release of trapped energy, in effect giving us back our lives. When we refuse to let go of trauma, a great deal of energy becomes bottled up—energy that we need if we are to transcend what has happened. By refusing to forgive, we are denied the opportunity to move into a new future.

Such an approach is exemplified by the life of Nelson Mandela, who, as we saw in chapter one, was imprisoned in South Africa for twenty-seven years. Had most of us found all these years of our life taken away from us, we would have come out of prison feeling victimized and enraged. But Mandela didn't plunge into resentment and bitterness during his years in prison. Instead he reflected on the situation in South Africa and came to the conclusion that only reconciliation could pave the way into a meaningful future. He came out of prison with a vision for his country because he was willing to go deeply into the prison experience instead of trying to push it away. The experience had changed his consciousness, and now he set about changing the consciousness of his nation to one of acceptance and reconciliation instead of resentment.

We can all see the need to let go, and yet so often we refuse to do so. How do we get beyond our egotistical refusal to let go and move on?

We are faced with the paradox of being part reflective human and part animal instinct. On the one hand, the ego refuses to let go of the past because to do so feels equivalent to a second injury or death experience. To let go, we have to re-experience the painful memories, which we have no doubt been attempting to block. Remembering forces us to face our fragility, vulnerability, and precarious position on this planet. To recognize how contingent our lives are at any given moment involves a shattering of the illusion of the permanence of our self-identity, and often the destruction of our entire belief system.

On the other hand, we are compelled biologically to rid ourselves of anything that obstructs our growth. We have an instinctual mechanism genetically encoded in us to help us let go of the old and begin something new. This ability to let go only seems to kick in when we diminish the ego's resistance and focus on the body's natural biological instincts.

Recall that Friedrich Nietzsche said we possess "the power to grow uniquely from within, to transform and incorporate the past and the unknown, to heal wounds, to replace what is lost, and to duplicate shattered structures from within."

Forgiving and letting go assure our unending evolution. Increasing our ability to feel our biological urge to heal allows the life force to work in us with less constraint.

FORGIVENESS MAY NOT COME EASILY

Since many of us find it difficult to forgive, it may be helpful for me to share my own experience of learning to forgive. One of the greatest challenges I encountered when recovering from post-traumatic stress was how to forgive those who I believed had harmed me. I felt like a victim. I was unable to forgive either God, nature, or the universe for what felt to me like betrayal. How could I forgive God, nature, or the universe for abandoning me when I needed them most?

Another aspect of learning to forgive involved the realization that I had put myself into extremely dangerous situations. I had made these choices willingly—no one forced them on me. How could I forgive myself for the pain I had brought on myself?

The post-traumatic stress I was suffering also affected other people in my life. Because of it I was enraged at myself and at life, but this wasn't other people's fault. Somehow I needed to forgive myself for my angry and violent behavior toward others.

How to forgive in each of these dimensions of life was a puddle of confusion in my mind, yet the underlying need to forgive was a recurring feeling.

I began my exploration of the concept of forgiveness cautiously. I already knew that trying to forgive in response to religious dictates wasn't going to work for me. I needed to explore the capacity for forgiveness as a natural aspect of our humanity. I was in search of a quality that plumbs the depths of what it means to be human, making possible a level of forgiveness that transcends religious and cultural influences.

It was important to me to understand whether the capacity for forgiveness is inherent in our humanity, and perhaps even part of our evolutionary process. I needed to know that the act of forgiving was not simply for the purpose of appeasing my guilt—although this might have been reason enough to forgive. I wanted to know whether forgiveness somehow enriches us as individuals, as well as enriching humanity as a whole.

My struggle to learn how to forgive lasted several years. Although I knew my inability to forgive was imprisoning me, I also knew that trying to hurry this delicate process would simply wound me all over again. However, as I slowly entered upon the process of letting go of my rage, anger, hurt, and sense of betrayal, forgiveness seemed to seep into my psyche and also my body. I found myself relaxing into being more human, which allowed a softness to return to me. As this happened, I found myself able to reach out to others with greater caring and concern for their suffering.

In his book *On Forgiveness*, Richard Holloway explains that forgiveness not only removes "dead weight from our past and gives us back our lives," but "the real beauty of forgiveness is that it can deliver the future to us."[17] This is what was happening in me. As I was able to forgive the perpetrators of the suffering I experienced—to forgive myself, God, and the universe—I found myself being delivered from the state of being frozen in the past into a future I could embrace with vision and hope. It was only then that my life could move forward with renewed vigor.

I eventually realized that the purpose of forgiveness isn't to let someone "off the hook." Forgiveness allows us to let go of something that is obstructing our growth. Each slow and painful step created a deeper realization that forgiveness is a fundamental process of human evolution from which the entire human community stands to benefit. I began to see that my individual attempts at forgiveness somehow contributed to the "evolution of the moral universe."[18]

Because it serves this purpose, forgiveness is not only an attractive quality but also a desirable goal. Only now do I realize that, without having gone through this process of learning to forgive, I would have remained confined in a form of psychic imprisonment that would still be dominating not only my life but the evolution of human morality. This is a beautiful and profound process that is worth being a part of.

"I WAS MORE TERRIFIED AND ANGRY THAN MY FAMILY"

I was working with a group of Eritrean refugees in Ethiopia who had not been able to contact or visit their families for several months because of intense fighting. They had no idea whether their family members were alive or in what conditions they may be living.

These people were full of anxiety, anger, fear, and despair. With each radio and television broadcast, they could only imagine the worst.

Finally the fighting ceased and they were able to visit their families. When they arrived, they were astonished at the stories of hardship they heard and the numerous near-death experiences their families went through during the intense fighting. Yet the family members who had endured the fighting were less disturbed than the ones who only imagined what their families must have endured.

Why were those who imagined the suffering more bitter, resentful, and less willing to resign themselves to their inevitable fate as war refugees? How is it that those who experienced the war were more positive, less fatalistic, and able to accept what had happened to them?

The explanation for this is that the ones who experienced the war were resigned to the fact that their belongings would be destroyed, while they were simultaneously elated at successfully struggling through the fighting.

The reality-based group had bodily sensations of aliveness, elation, comfort, and safety as a result of surviving their ordeal. These physical sensations helped temper the imagination and put their experience in perspective.

The other group's imagination generated a horrifying illusion that was completely divorced from the body's senses, and therefore only partially informed by reality.

It's common for people who haven't experienced the same trauma as their loved ones to be even more bitter, fearful, resentful, and vengeful than the person who endured and survived the trauma. Imagination is powerful—which can make it dangerous if it isn't connected to the body's actual experience.

It also turns out that those who suffer can forgive more readily than those who only participate in suffering through their imagination. It's easier to forgive because one's suffering is informed by reality.

Refusing to let go of the past traps us in a neural feedback loop that causes the trauma to be replayed over and over in our minds in an endless cycle of madness. Eventually the neurological process within our brain will transform this chaos into ideations of hate, revenge, shame, depression, and in some cases suicide.

Once we enter this arena we can be trapped forever in the compulsive vengeance mentality of a victim, rather than enjoying the freedom that flows from the forgiveness of a survivor.

TAKE RESPONSIBILITY FOR YOUR WELLBEING

In the end, letting go of the past is the responsibility of each trauma survivor. It's each individual's responsibility to guarantee that revenge doesn't rob them of their future.

When violence broke out in India toward the end of British rule, Gandhi was far away. But he felt a call to return home and wade into the very heart of the violence. When he ended up in prison he used the time to reflect on the violence. Through his reflection he came to a great insight—that violence cannot be ended with violence but must be actively met with nonviolence. It was a new level of consciousness, achieved by embracing his situation, not evading it. And so he was able to let go of the need for revenge and to inspire many to do the same.

Once we determine to let go, our natural instinct for survival is so powerful that it transcends our need to entertain hatred or thoughts of revenge. As Peter Levine discovered, "A person who has successfully renegotiated a traumatic event is transformed by the experience, and feels no need for revenge—shame and blame dissolve in the powerful wake of renewal and self-acceptance."[19]

To let go of the effects of a traumatic experience is to unlock ourselves from the past and prepare for our next evolutionary experience. Trauma in this light becomes not just an integral part of our journey but the way we learn to be fully developed people. We discover that on the other end of a frightening episode, we have greater maturity, compassion, and wisdom.

16

Tough Times Can Make You Stronger

❀ ❀ ❀ ❀ ❀

WITH OUR RECOVERY FROM EACH TRAUMATIC EPISODE, we give into and accept more easily the way our life has unfolded. Paradoxically, the more we let ourselves flow with life's tides, the more we discover how to take control of our life and invest ourselves more fully than ever in the precariousness of being human.

Researchers conducted an experiment with three sets of chicks. The first group of chicks formed the control group. This group received no intervention on the part of the researchers. The second group was held in the hands of the researchers until they experienced the freeze response. This group was then released and the chicks were allowed to recover, which involved going through trembling and fluttering their feathers. The third set of chicks was likewise held in the hands of the researchers to evoke the freeze response. But when they were released and began to tremor, they were again held to prevent the tremoring process from occurring.

When the second set of chicks, which had been traumatized and allowed to discharge the trauma, were placed in a vat of water to see how long they could swim before reaching the point of drowning, they turned out to have even greater endurance than the first set of chicks, which hadn't been traumatized at all. In other words, the traumatized chicks that were allowed to discharge the trauma had become *more resilient.*

The third group, which didn't discharge the trauma, sank to the bottom of the vat without attempting to swim. They had learned to be helpless in the face of a threat.

Through the unending cycle of trauma recovery, the human species also learns how to adapt to life-threatening situations. This process of adaptation makes humanity as a whole stronger and smarter in the face of future challenges. If we didn't possess this evolutionary instinct, we would have died out as a species shortly after we emerged on the planet.

MAKING SENSE OF TRAUMATIC TIMES

Accepting trauma as a natural part of life allows us to see such times in a new light.

When we experience one of life's painful events it initially feels unbearable. The experience often overwhelms our entire sense of self. Any ideas we may have held of there being some kind of logic to life can be shattered. Indeed, we often wonder if we will ever recover from such pain and disruption.

The self-renewal that happens in the recovery process occurs because we are forced to explore painful depths we wouldn't otherwise have chosen to experience. Whether we like it or not, whether we want to or not, our recovery process forces us deeper into our body and further into serious reflection than we would normally dare to go.

As painful as this exploration may be, in the end we have to resign ourselves to the fact that, as one observer put it, "this is the way things are," and they have been made this way "by factors that are not in the person's control."[20]

This depth of inner exploration inevitably creates a deeper sense of connectedness to our personal life, together with stronger bonds of connectedness to others and even the universe. In other words, it is precisely the shattering effect of trauma that forces us to think in new ways, feel at deeper levels, and relate to others more compassionately.

MOTHER TERESA SHINES A LIGHT

"How do you deal with trauma?" I asked Mother Teresa, who we saw in chapter one was made stronger by trauma. She had experienced a lot of trauma during her childhood due to social and political hardships in Skopje (now the republic of Macedonia). She also encountered endless trauma on the streets of India.

Mother told me, "I was on a spiritual retreat, trying to decide what to do about the severe poverty I saw in India." She belonged to a financially comfortable religious community and couldn't equate living in such a community with what she saw on the streets. "I gained little insight from the retreat," she confessed, "but on the train on my way back to Calcutta, staring out the window daydreaming, it came to me what I had to do."

I leaned forward in my chair, waiting to hear the wisdom that would flow from this inspiring woman. "It was one of those moments when you finally let go and you stop thinking and stop praying," she said. "At such a moment, something just comes to you."

Mother paused, then smiled. "What came to me was the simple insight, 'Don't let people die alone.'"

That's all Mother Teresa had in terms of a vision. She went back to her religious community and simply said, "I need to go hold people so they don't die alone." Initially, she had no pretensions of starting a religious community, simply the imperative to embrace people's trauma rather than push it away because it was repulsive.

Mother Teresa could have been bitter about her childhood hardships. Instead, she allowed them to touch her soul and raise her consciousness, moving her to reach out to the sick and dying of India with deep compassion.

Most people push trauma away because they are afraid of it. It's too intense for them. But Mother Teresa actually embraced trauma when it came into her life, allowing it to transform her consciousness, seeing it as a path to a deeper spirituality.

Mother Teresa not only embraced the trauma in her life, she actually went out and sought traumatized people to help. She knew that working with the poorest of the poor would deepen her spiritually.

If most of us seek out trauma situations in which to help, it's usually because we feel guilty. Few of us go out to live in trauma in order to allow it to change us. This is what separated Mother from the rest of us. It didn't matter if it was a flood, an earthquake, or a rape, Mother Teresa saw in all of the suffering she dealt with a potential for spiritual awakening. While most of us try to push trauma away, she embraced it.

How was she able to love the filthy, starving people who were dying in the streets? The answer lies in how she viewed them. In her words, "I see everyone as Jesus." This terminology comes from her particular religious tradition, but it simply points to the fact that she saw every person as a sacred being. She reached out to them easily and readily because of who she saw them to be. She didn't care about getting herself dirty and she ignored the stench. She treated each person as an individual of enormous potential who was on a spiritual path. Because of this, she could love each and every one of them. If we also saw all humans as sacred, we would want to get down on the ground and embrace them too.

TRAUMA AS OUR TEACHER

Trauma has the ability to teach us what love is, while simultaneously bringing out our innate capacity for deep caring. Through traumatic experiences, we can discover our true mettle as compassionate individuals.

Such a discovery about ourselves changes how we live our ordinary, everyday lives. For instance, after the Twin Towers collapsed, many moved out of New York, back to their hometown. They moved not because they were afraid, but because they came to the realization that playing with their children and being around their extended family was more important than the riches they were accumulating in the Big Apple. The trauma of 9/11 opened their hearts to a deeper appreciation of life and a more important way to spend their few years on this planet.

A year after 9/11 people frequently commented to me that the event had changed their life. They didn't want the trauma they went through, but since it happened, they allowed it to change them.

People who have healed successfully from trauma discover that their life is richer, fuller, and more caring than they experienced before. This is what the evolution of the human species is about. The development of compassion, caring, and sensitivity to the pain of humanity emerges as a result of recovering from our own painful experience of life.

TRUST IN THE GOODNESS OF LIFE

Our era is witnessing tremendous suffering on a global scale. It seems impossible to arrest such suffering despite our desire to do so. In light of this unstoppable, irreversible, and in many ways self-destructive period in our history, we need to ask what good can come of all this pain.

When trauma occurs on a large scale, can we trust that the universe is helping humans evolve into a more ethical, moral, and caring species?

Although traumatic experiences are increasing on our planet, these experiences may be triggering an expansion of human consciousness and compassion. As more and more people approach the trauma that comes into their life as a way of growing instead of trying to push it away, they are discovering the deep hidden message it has for humanity.

While changing planes at the airport in Phoenix, Arizona, I had a little time before my flight to Africa, so visited a small aerospace museum. I was stunned by a quote from one of the astronauts. In essence he said, "On the first day in space, we were all pointing out our countries. On the second day in space, we were all pointing out our continents. On the third day, we were all pointing out our planet."

How wonderful it would be if we could all have the experience of looking at our planet from a distance and seeing that all humans are a single species dependent on one another for our survival and continued evolution. I have a hunch that the escalating trauma on our planet is pushing us to embrace just such a viewpoint!

It's fascinating to see how many movie and music stars are reaching out to Third World cultures. As these stars visit countries that are in trauma, they find themselves reflecting on their experience of people's suffering, and this causes a shift in their consciousness. They realize that it's unacceptable for humans to live this way, and in turn they seek to raise our awareness of the need to help such societies heal themselves.

If we accept trauma as an intrinsic aspect of life, the period we are passing through on Earth at the moment can be viewed as the pain of the human species going through another birthing process, this time in order to be born into a new era of human consciousness.

Such a heightened state of consciousness is desperately needed right now. Einstein recognized that, with the splitting of the atom, our technology had advanced further than our moral and ethical ability to handle such power. The global trauma we are experiencing may be a way for our species to develop the moral and ethical dimensions necessary to responsibly handle our technological advancement.

NO WAY BUT FORWARD

Once a trauma befalls us, we have no option but to follow its life-altering path. At times, this path passes through the black night of helplessness and hopelessness. It can terrify us by unveiling the fragility, precariousness, and vulnerability of our humanity. It tears at the very fabric of our identity and radically redefines our view of life.

It's precisely because this experience has burned the bridges of our past ways of thinking that we embark upon a new way of being in life. The old ways of thinking and relating no longer suffice, and a new way begins to reveal itself.

People who consciously journey through the life-altering experience of a traumatic event seem to reintegrate and re-embody themselves in such a way that they are more receptive to an expanded, more cosmic experience of life than was previously available to them. Trauma is thus the universe's way of helping humanity to mature into a wiser, more compassionate state that honors our inherent oneness.

17

A Soldier Shows the Way

❀ ❀ ❀ ❀ ❀

ONE OF THE SADDEST AND MOST EMOTIONALLY PAINFUL EXPERIENCES is to have a loved one commit suicide. The haunting questions of, "What could I have done to help? Why didn't I see it coming? Why did this happen?" can persist for years or even a lifetime. A great deal of judging and blaming often follows in the wake of a suicide.

Fortunately I have never had a client commit suicide, although I have dealt with many suicidal clients. After working with numerous people who have contemplated suicide, I realized that suicidal individuals exhibit a common pattern of behavior in their *body,* not just in their psyche.

"EVEN DEATH WAS BETTER THAN THIS INNER NUMBNESS"

A young soldier I was working with had witnessed some truly inhuman sights during his time in battle. I met him about a year after he had left the military, at a point in his life when he was suicidal.

This young man couldn't stand living with his memories. Even though he only saw the sights that so shocked him one time, he replayed the scenario relentlessly in his mind until, as he told me, "I have seen those sights over a thousand times."

I inquired, "How is your body handling these memories?"

"I have always just numbed out," he admitted. "That way, I don't feel anything inside. I don't feel my own self, and I don't feel any connection to other people. I am completely alone both inside and out."

"So, what do you do when you feel sadness or anger?" I asked.

"When I get any feelings, I numb out," he explained. "If the feelings are too strong to numb them, I will take drugs or get drunk to guarantee I get rid of them."

This soldier's insight into himself later led me to question how much of a role the body plays when people contemplate suicide. Coming from a body-oriented background, I began to question why psychotherapy hasn't attempted to explain thoughts of suicide in terms of a physical response as well as a psychological one.

It's already recognized that, as a living organism, the human body pulsates with a genetic encoding that compels it to live life to its fullest, just like any other plant or animal on the planet. So what happens when an individual deadens their ability to feel the natural impulse to live?

Numbing of the body during the onslaught of a trauma is a natural protective mechanism. The continuation of this numbing after the trauma has ended is where the danger lies. If we deliberately continue to numb the body from pain, we are also numbing our ability to feel the natural pulsation of life in our body.

Through the insight of this soldier, I stumbled upon the fact that when bodywork accompanies the counseling of a suicidal individual, the person is often able to increase internal sensation and feel the natural pulsation to live, thereby decreasing the mind's thoughts of dying.

"I AM STILL ALIVE!"

Research has demonstrated that we possess the capacity to communicate with and receive communication from our internal bodily systems.

The unconscious mind actually has a physiological center, which is an extension of our nervous system, and this physiological center supplies information to the brain. The brain must feel an appropriate amount of stimulation from the body to function properly. If the brain lacks input from the body, it creates its own. In such a situation, the mind begins to make the imagination seem real. If that imagination is terrifying, grotesque, or horrifying, the body will continue to numb itself to escape this overwhelming input from the mind.

When this occurs, the images in the mind become stronger than the pulsation of the living organism. The mind can then override the body's encoding to live. In other words, the increase in suicidal thoughts is directly connected to the decrease in physical sensation, while the decrease in physical sensation contributes to the increase in suicidal tendencies.

With this understanding of the mind's ability to disconnect from the body, I decided to include bodywork with counseling of suicidal clients. I discovered that the deeper and more intense the bodywork, the more connected individuals felt to their body and subsequently to me. Such people couldn't believe that someone was able to connect with them despite their overwhelming feeling of aloneness.

Clients described this connection as "a good feeling." It caused them to realize, as one person put it, that "deep inside, under the pain and numbness, I am still alive."

With each session, I continued working with the body and also gave homework assignments designed to stimulate positive bodily sensations. Gradually the person's ability to feel their natural body's genetic encoding *to live* became stronger than the ego's imagination that they needed to die.

I believe it's not only possible but also advantageous to capitalize on the psycho-physical connection when working with suicidal tendencies. Physical intervention coupled with psychological counseling offers a more holistic resolution for suicidal thoughts than the traditional psychological approach. It's a combination that has the power to derail the seemingly one-track mind of suicidal individuals.

SLEEPWALKING THROUGH LIFE

Wrote T.S. Eliot, "We shall not cease from exploration, and the end of all exploring will be to arrive where we started and know the place for the first time."

I don't know a better description of what trauma can do for us. Eliot is describing a state in which we are fully present, so that we are truly aware of what is going on both within ourselves and all around us. It's a state in which we are here, now, giving our full attention to the life we are living.

This isn't the usual state of humans. Instead of being fully alive, many of us sleepwalk through our day, which is at best punctuated with brief moments of real awareness. Much of the time we go through the motions—in our relationships, our work, our social and leisure activities. We are here, but not *really* here—much as we often drive a stretch of road and can't remember driving it.

The human tendency to escape from awareness is enshrined in the misunderstanding of religious traditions that focus on avoidance of much of this life, or that emphasize an afterlife. To be "detached" from life is thought by many to be a spiritual achievement. Joseph Campbell recognized the folly of this when he said that enlightenment is the opposite of what most think. To be enlightened isn't to experience an absence of feeling, but to be deeply involved in every aspect of our lives. "Non-attachment" simply means that we don't derive our *identity* from the people and things around us, but from our own deep core.

There is a sense in which all of us need to experience suicide—not the death of our body and spirit, but the death of the inauthentic way we live our lives so much of the time. We need to detach from all that isn't truly who we are and that doesn't serve our real identity, which is far deeper than the person we tend to imagine we are as a result of growing up in families and a culture that in so many ways inadvertently shut off our awareness of our essence.

When trauma comes into our life, it can put us in touch with the depth dimension of reality, our true being. It can put an end to life in the impoverished way we have been living it. It stops us from skating along on the surface of everyday events, inviting us to go deeper into our life.

When we connect with the depth dimension of existence, we experience the essence of people, events, things, and places, instead of just their appearance. In such a state our windows of perception are wide open, our consciousness fully attuned, our attention focused so that we are absorbing what we are involved in.

The phenomenon I am referring to is *transcendent* but *not transcendental*. It isn't an awareness of planes of reality beyond this reality, but rather involves full and complete immersion in our present life. It's an experience of transparency, where we see to the heart of something—into our own heart, and subsequently into the hearts of others.

All sorts of elaborate religious and philosophical systems have been developed to help us become aware. But when they are misunderstood, they can take us away from being fully actualized individuals. Often they make it appear difficult to become actualized, as if it were a process that requires years if not lifetimes. The power of trauma is that is has the ability to jolt us awake and capture our full attention in an instant.

Systems devised to deliver us into a fullness of being generally advocate a certain protocol. There is a particular way of looking, a way of talking, a way of walking, even. In contrast, trauma blasts its way into our lives, replacing protocol with pain that can't be ignored. In so doing, it elicits realness from us. Pretense goes out the window as reality rushes in.

None of us likes to be confronted with the truth about ourselves because our ego—the person we think of ourselves as being, based on the way we were brought up to see ourselves—doesn't want to recognize how we are short-changing ourselves on joy. We resist breaking out of our mediocrity. But when trauma strikes, we have a chance to question and to face up to why we settle for a surface existence. The pressure and the heat of the situation crack open the shell of our learned way of being, opening us up to our authentic being and full presence in everything we do.

So it is that we return to the ordinary events of everyday life, but now we know them for the first time. We have become wise, able to appreciate the whole of life for the wondrous adventure it is when lived in the present moment.

18

The Body and the Present Moment

꽃 꽃 꽃 꽃 꽃

"AT EVERY STAGE OF HUMAN DEVELOPMENT," someone once said, "the greatest ally we have is the body because it forces us to live fully in the present moment!"

One of the amazing aspects of engaging in bodywork is that the body is a pure history book of what has happened to it. This is because, unlike the ego, it cannot make things up. What it tells us about ourselves is pure and undistorted.

For instance, the body only contracts when there is something it perceives as dangerous. It doesn't simply wake up one morning and say, "I think I will contract today." It only contracts or distorts the natural rate at which it vibrates when a particular experience seems to warrant such a change.

TREMORS AND THE BODY'S HISTORY

When I work with a client's body, I am aware that everything—every emotion, feeling, or physical sensation emanating from the individual's body—is revealing an accurate history of what the body has experienced.

When the body begins to tremor, it releases chronic tension. Through this release process, the body tells its story. The places where the tremors move through, along with the places where they are unable to move through the body, reveal the physical aspects of the body's history. Which emotions are released and which are not released reveals the specific emotional aspects of these experiences. The memories or thoughts that are evoked by the tremors reveal the cognitive aspects of these same experiences.

The body is unveiling each aspect of its history when it is tremoring.

SPIRITUALITY THROUGH THE BODY

All spiritual practices emphasize that in order to connect with the spiritual dimension of ourselves, we must live in the present moment.

If you have ever had a really good massage, you know what this feels like. You might go to your massage therapist with complaints of muscle aches and pains from having a tense week. If the massage successfully releases tight muscles, the stress you are carrying also releases. Now you can take a deep breath and actually experience yourself as more fully alive, more fully present. Perhaps you comment, "Wow, that was great. I was able to let go of everything I have been carrying around for the past week."

Through the release of tight muscles, you were able to let go of the past and came more fully into the present moment. And this present moment feels more alive, more relaxed, safer, and more comfortable.

Living in the present moment is actually the safest and most comfortable place we can exist. For instance, when I was living in war zones, I experienced less anxiety when I remained in the present moment—even during bombings. It was the terror from the past and the anticipation of future uncontrollable experiences that provoked anxiety. Somehow I felt more in control when I focused on the present moment, even though nothing had actually changed in my external circumstances. The past and future seemed completely out of my control and therefore more terrifying.

During my fifteen years of using the Trauma Release Process™ in nineteen countries with thousands of people who have experienced severe trauma, I was slowly and almost imperceptibly invited to see how the tremors themselves create a deeper awareness of our inner self. This awareness is intricately connected to the emergence of our spiritual self, which is our true self.

This process of deepening spiritual awareness began to reveal itself to me as people shared with me the spiritual experiences they were having as a result of allowing the tremors to relax their body.

As a result of these stories, I began reading spiritual literature and exploring the spiritual journeys of the people in the war-torn countries where I was living. Many common themes and ideas began to surface, which spanned the different cultures and countries. I was gradually able to piece together the insights that had accumulated in these cultures and been preserved in a variety of religious traditions. Reflecting on my experience of the Trauma Release Process™ in light of my own spiritual process, these diverse cultural expressions began to form a picture.

TREMORS AND THE BODY

All along we have seen that tremors are a natural mechanism of the body, intended to relax muscle tissue. They are encoded in our DNA. We are genetically encoded to tremor. The exercises do not do anything to the body except reawaken and reengage this natural tremoring mechanism that has been dormant inside us.

All our life long it's been natural for our muscles to contract because of dangers the body-mind felt it needed to protect itself from. But when this tension isn't released and hence becomes chronic, it prevents the body from being fully alive in the present. Its ability to express its organic liveliness is restricted by the patterns of muscle tension. When the body is allowed to tremor, the tremors release this tension, thereby allowing the body to come more fully into the present moment.

This is how I have been able to understand the tremors as an access point into the spiritual body of the individual. As we begin to tremor, we experience the inner energy field of the body. Since the tremors are being evoked by an instinctual part of the brain—the brain stem, rather than the more conscious part of the brain, the neocortex—the individual's consciousness shifts from perceiving the body purely as a dense physical structure to experiencing it as a living organism. This is often the first time many of us have been able to gain access to our inner energetic field, which we now experience as alive and connected to the universe.

Babbett Rothschild commented, "One only has to read the most basic of the literature on the function of the brain, the nervous system and the physiology of stress to understand that the mind and the body are undeniably linked."[21]

The initial awareness that accompanies access to our inner energetic field triggers a paradigm shift in our consciousness. The sense of our individuality and our separateness from others is radically challenged by the experience of these tremors. As we continue to repeat the tremoring exercises, we reinforce this new paradigm of self. Each time the denser body-self releases its tension through tremoring, our true vibrational frequency grows stronger.

As we experience a shift in our consciousness, our energy level, and our vibrational frequency, it produces a sense of lightness in the physical body, greater clarity about our true self, and a more obvious connectedness to others.

This became clear to me in a workshop I was giving with a group of highly sensitized yoga practitioners. As they were lying on the floor tremoring, they realized that their individual tremors were somehow connecting to others who were lying on the floor tremoring. At one point, one of the participants remarked, "It actually feels like we are one vibrating organism. We aren't separate. It's as though our individual vibrational fields have expanded to become one large vibrational field of which we are all a part." This observation was quickly accepted and agreed upon by the other participants.

After the experience was over, the group reflected on what it felt like to achieve a collective vibratory rate in which everyone experienced a sense of oneness, while simultaneously experiencing a heightened sense of their individuality. Their reflections were consistent with those of many who describe the paradox of being a separate person and yet a part of the collective whole.

One of the yoga practitioners commented, "This experience was both paradoxical and transformative. It was paradoxical in that I felt more like myself than ever before, while at the same time I felt like my individual identity was completely connected to the oneness of the universe. In other words, I was more myself and less myself at the same time."

Another participant related, "During this experience, I couldn't understand or explain the experience at all, and yet it feels like it all made sense to me." She continued, "Although I don't know how to talk about this experience, I still feel compelled to talk about it."

One participant asked how long they had been lying on the floor tremoring. Why did he want to know? He explained, "Once we felt ourselves tremoring as one large vibrational field, time seemed to vanish. We could have been there one minute or one hour. I couldn't tell and it didn't matter. It could have been an instant or an eternity. It all seemed to blend together."

Another participant shared that although he was aware I was walking around the room, he seemed to be both unaware of others in the room and yet fully in touch with everything that was happening.

As I traveled from country to county, I was forced to change my terminology so each of the different cultures could embrace the concept of spirituality. In order not to alienate people who didn't identify with the word spiritual, I instead spoke of a "peak experience."

As I asked people about the peak experiences of their life, I was astonished at the similarity as well as the simplicity of these experiences. People in many different cultures described what happened during these peak moments. Despite cultural, religious, or spiritual differences, the same two aspects stood out as emerged from the yoga practitioners: The experiences were both *transformative* and *paradoxical*.

TREMORS AND CONSCIOUSNESS

The Trauma Release Process™ can help create a shift in consciousness. It affords us an experience of our body as a living organism that has needs and behaviors not under our conscious control.

The vibration created during the exercises presents us with an opportunity to access the place where matter interfaces with pure energy. This is what allows a shift in consciousness to get underway. A new paradigm of our own existence begins to emerge, and we experience what it's like to live in commonality with all other living organisms on the planet. The tremors help dissolve our sensation of separateness, birthing in us a new sense of oneness.

Tremoring helps us reconnect with our essential being in the present moment because nothing past or future disturbs the organism as it vibrates to its aliveness. Tremors only operate in the here and now.

TREMORS AND PHYSICS

Reading current literature on physics one day, I realized that, like all organisms, the human body vibrates at a certain frequency. This means that the human body has a naturally healthy vibratory rate.

The body's natural vibratory frequency becomes distorted and diminished by the accumulation of tension patterns. This is often why we may feel sluggish and lifeless, or anxious and nervous, when tension builds in the body. Our vibratory frequency is being distorted, which causes us to feel disconnected from ourselves as well as from the universe.

Tremoring dissolves interfering tension patterns, allowing the body to restore itself back to its healthy vibratory frequency. When this occurs, we feel reconnected with not only ourselves but also the universe. This sense of reconnection is like, "Wow, life feels great. I feel connected. Even when things may not appear to be going well, life is somehow less threatening." Through these tremors, we access our inherent inner peace, because the mind, which is so often preoccupied with either the past or the future, has been quieted by relaxing the body—and the body exists only in the present moment.

The closer we are to our natural vibratory rate, the less disconnected we feel. In psychological terms, the ego of separateness recedes into the background, and the spiritual awareness that we are a living organism connected to all other living organisms comes to the foreground.

Feeling connected to the universe is a much safer feeling than the isolation and loneliness of individuality and separateness. The present moment holds the key to our liberation into a fully alive experience of our humanity, for we can't find the present moment as long as we are trapped in our thoughts. We must come into the here and now. Tremoring helps us become present since it's a bodily activity, and the present is the only time frame in which the body can exist.

Because these tremors are so natural for the body, when they begin to occur the body recognizes its true nature. However, the mind will often wonder what's happening. The mind perceives tremors as strange and unnatural—in fact, possibly a sign of weakness and fearfulness, and certainly embarrassing. But tremors cause the mind to recognize it is encased in a living organism that has a spontaneous ability to restore itself to health. This causes a shift in our self-identity and increases our level of consciousness. Prior to such a shift, we had lost our reference point.

Once when I was giving a workshop, an Asian woman and I got into a conversation about the pelvis, in which lies the center of gravity of the body. She explained, "In eastern traditions, the life force of the body is located in the pelvis. This energy is referred to by different names such as hara, chi, or prana." She went on to tell me that in the Japanese tradition, if a person commits suicide, they do this by performing hari-kari. This is the process of running a sword through the lower belly. It is believed that by doing this, the individual kills their spirit. With great insight and simplicity, she explained, "When people in the western world commit suicide, they most often shoot themselves in the head." This, she said, is where westerners think their life force exists. She was absolutely correct. The western world tends to be so mind-oriented, we feel it's our mind that's driving us crazy—and consequently imagine that the only way out of our craziness is to kill the mind. It doesn't seem to occur to people in the West that a better way out of this feeling is to return to the present moment, to which the body offers access.

A wonderful result of reactivating the tremoring mechanism is that tremors begin occurring spontaneously each time we find ourselves in a stressful or traumatic situation. The ability to tremor with each highly charged event allows the body to discharge the excessively high energetic charges connected with distressing events. It's a wonderful thing to know that our body will automatically begin to restore itself anytime we find ourselves in a distressing situation in the future. The implication is that no amount of stress or trauma in the future can cause long-term damaging effects. We can experience a traumatic event and shortly afterwards begin the natural restoration process, so that we no longer have to carry the experience around in our body for years afterwards.

PART II

The Trauma Release Process (TRP)™

19

The Trauma Release Process™

❀ ❀ ❀ ❀ ❀

WE TURN NOW TO THE TRAUMA RELEASE PROCESS™ itself. The exercises are not only for people who have been greatly traumatized, but are intended to be helpful to all of us.

I came up with the exercises as a result of living and working in traumatizing situations for years. I wasn't trying to develop any kind of technique. The trauma affected my body, and I simply reflected on what it did to me. From the reflection came the exercises.

All of us have the potential to improve the quality of our life in the wake of trauma. Whether this happens or not depends on whether we go into the trauma and reflect on it, or whether we push it away because it's too painful.

The following exercises enable us to go into our trauma by means of our body. As we perform them, we revisit the traumatic patterns established in our body, which enables us to release them. In the process of the release, a new consciousness is born.

Most other exercises are designed to release surface level tension in the body. This is insufficient for dealing with the deep chronic tension generated by trauma. Oftentimes these milder forms of exercise leave the individual feeling helpless and confused when the exercises fail to relieve the tension. What is needed is a process whereby the individual uses the body's natural shaking mechanism to release deep trauma tension patterns.

The Trauma Release Process™, although simple and painless, is specifically designed to evoke the body's shaking mechanism, thereby releasing the deep, chronic muscle contractions created by severe shock or trauma. Used regularly, it can also prevent life's everyday minor stresses from turning into chronic tension.

The exercises are designed to stress the seven thigh flexor muscles commonly referred to as hip flexors. These exercises rely purely on the body's natural ability to trigger tremors. Rather than focusing on specific muscle tension patterns established during a particular stressful event, the exercises address a generic pattern of muscle tension in the body. By using the body's natural muscle tremor process, they relax all muscle patterns associated with stress.

The key to these exercises is their ability to evoke shaking from the center of gravity of the body located in the pelvis, using nothing but the natural mechanism of the body. When shaking is evoked at this powerful center, it reverberates throughout the entire body, seeking out any deep chronic tension that lies in its path and naturally discharging this tension and relaxing the muscles. Tremors will initially begin in the upper thighs and work their way into the psoas muscles. The shaking will then travel through the pelvis, into the lower back, and finally up the spine into the shoulders, neck, arms, and hands. Each time you do the exercises, the shaking pattern may change, and various types of shaking can occur.

If for any reason you feel the need to stop the exercises or the shaking, simply do so by stretching your legs out flat onto the floor and relaxing on your back or curling up on your side. As always, the key is to respect your body, emotions, and psyche. You can always return to the exercises when you feel calm, safe, and comfortable.

The only thing these exercises do is to release deep chronic tension in the muscle tissue. However, if you have been using this tension to protect yourself throughout most of your life, releasing it could evoke the original anxiety and fear that created the tension in the first place. Should you begin to experience such feelings, all you have to do is simply slow down the rate at which you are performing the exercises. In this way, you will learn how to continue releasing tension without evoking an overwhelming sense of fear or anxiety. This is a self-empowering experience, because you will learn that you can gradually replace your chronic tension without overwhelming yourself with unpleasant emotions.

If you have no emotional response to the exercises, this doesn't mean something is wrong. Simply enjoy the vibration caused by the exercises and continue to repeat them. They have a cumulative effect of relaxing the body at deeper and deeper levels. Many who have done extensive bodywork find the shaking to be a profound integrating tool for the psychosomatic work they have already completed.

For people who have experienced severe degrees of trauma, the trauma recovery process may seem daunting. These exercises, although simple and non-invasive, can have the effect of being overwhelming if the post-traumatic stress symptoms surface very quickly. The way to avoid this is to slow down the exercises to small periods of time. If the exercises cause emotions to surface, simply do them for a shorter time so that you can integrate the emotions in digestible amounts. In this way you can avoid sensations of emotional flooding or dissociating from the emotions.

It's similar to going on a rollercoaster ride. If you start with a rollercoaster that is too big, you will find yourself desperately squeezing the handlebar, holding on for dear life. However, if you begin on a smaller rollercoaster, you experience the dips with actual pleasure and excitement. The same is true of the rollercoaster of emotions. Simply allow the tremors to release only the amount of emotion that you can safely and comfortably integrate at the moment. Don't take on more than you can handle. There is no need to hurry the recovery process. Going faster than you can integrate the process will simply overwhelm you, which is exactly what a traumatic experience is—an overwhelming of your system. If you go slowly and steadily in your recovery process, it will take you on a remarkable journey that restores physical suppleness and emotional stability, as well as bring insights you never experienced before. By going at your own pace, you can experience your recovery as an amazing journey into one of life's most profound experiences.

HOW OFTEN?

Since the Trauma Release Process™ triggers responses that are natural to the body, in most cases the exercises can be practiced every day without harm. They can also be used simply for the purpose of relieving the tensions created from the daily stress of life.

The shaking may produce a feeling of exhaustion, as if you just finished a long workout. Or it may free up a lot of energy, so that you feel invigorated. Some find the exercises calming and therefore do them in the evening as a way of relaxing. Many who find them energizing do them in the morning or afternoon when they would like more energy.

It can be useful to incorporate these exercises into your regular exercise routine. Simply add another fifteen minutes onto the end of your workout so that you close with shaking. This will also relieve any stress created in the muscles as a result of your workout.

The rule of thumb is to follow the prompting of your body. As you become increasingly sensitive to your body, it will inform you of when you need to relieve stress.

If you don't have an intense adverse reaction to the exercises, you can practice them every other day for a month. Taking this approach helps to orient your body to the shaking and allows you to gradually decrease the tension in your body. After a month you can reduce the number of times you do the exercises to approximately twice a week. If you do them less than this, your body may once again begin to accumulate stress and tighten up.

Does the shaking ever stop? As long as you inhabit your body, you should be able to shake. It's a natural mechanism designed to relieve deep chronic tension. But once the deep tensions of the body are released and the deleterious effects of life's traumas and stresses have subsided, your body will simply produce a very fine tremor that feels a bit like a mild and pleasant electric current running throughout your entire organism.

YOUR TENSION IS UNIQUE TO YOU

Many clients say to me, "I wish I was shaking in a different way." Or, "I wish my back would shake." It's an error to wish your body would shake in any manner other than the way it does. The body shakes in the manner it needs to. The best advice is to never judge your body, just observe it. All the dialogue in the mind is simply ego interference.

If you find that your shaking is strong, it's an indicator that the large muscles in the body are breaking up iceberg-like tension in your muscles. Once your energy can flow more easily, this strong shaking will subside.

Sometimes you may find that strong shaking gives way to milder shaking, then returns. This is the body's way of systematically relieving the patterns of stress embedded in the muscles. Just allow your body to shake the way it needs to. It fully understands what it must do to dissolve the patterns of tension that have been created over the years.

Since each person has a unique set of experiences in life, we have all developed unique patterns of tension. We will each shake in different ways depending on our individual tension patterns and the readiness of our muscles to relax. Consequently, there is no one correct way of shaking. On the contrary, there are as many ways as there are bodies.

If you get more shaking in the standing position, should you stay there? If you get shaking while standing, and this feels more comfortable for you, then continue to stand and shake. Just remember that you may get the shaking in a different position each time you do the exercises. Eventually you should be able to get the shaking in a variety of positions. Each one has its own value.

A WORD OF CAUTION

The Trauma Release Process™ has been used safely and effectively by a wide variety of people around the world in many different situations. The tremors experienced in these exercises simply relax muscle tension patterns. Therefore, in most instances and for most people, the Trauma Release Process™ is safe when self-administered.

As already stated, in the process of relaxing deep chronic muscular tension, some individuals experience emotions that reflect the original cause of the creation of these tension patterns. Depending on the severity of the tension being released, the emotional discharge could range from mild to severe. For a minority of people, the exercises will be so effective in helping release trauma patterns in the body that their use may result in an intense and perhaps uncomfortable emotional experience. In such a situation, an individual may require the direct supervision and support of a health professional who has training and experience in this field.

Should you experience any physical or emotional discomfort upon using these exercises, please stop them and immediately consult a medical professional.

20

The Exercises

❁ ❁ ❁ ❁ ❁

To ACHIEVE THE BEST RESULTS FOR THESE EXERCISES, and to allow for greater movement in the feet and ankles, you may wish to remove your shoes and socks, unless this causes your feet to slide on the floor.

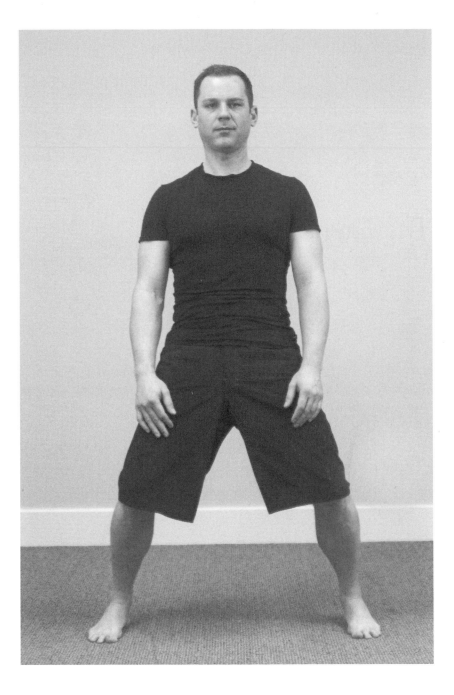

Exercise 1

step 1. Spread your feet shoulder width apart.

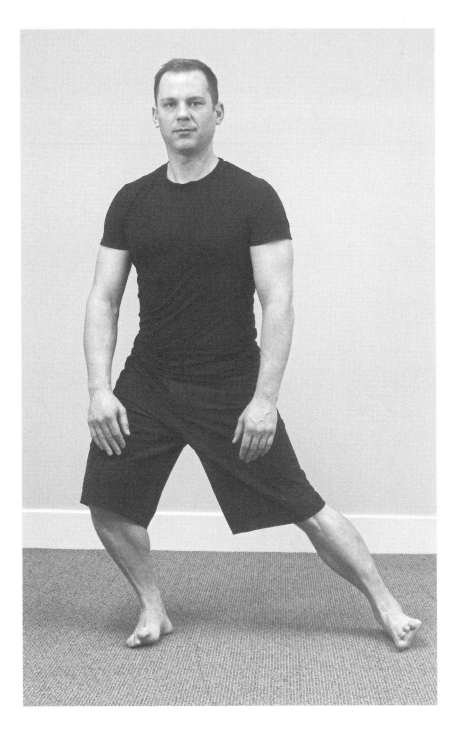

step 2. Slowly sway back and forth, turning both feet up onto one side in the same direction. This means you will stand on the outside of one foot and on the inside of the other foot. Hold this position for 15 seconds.

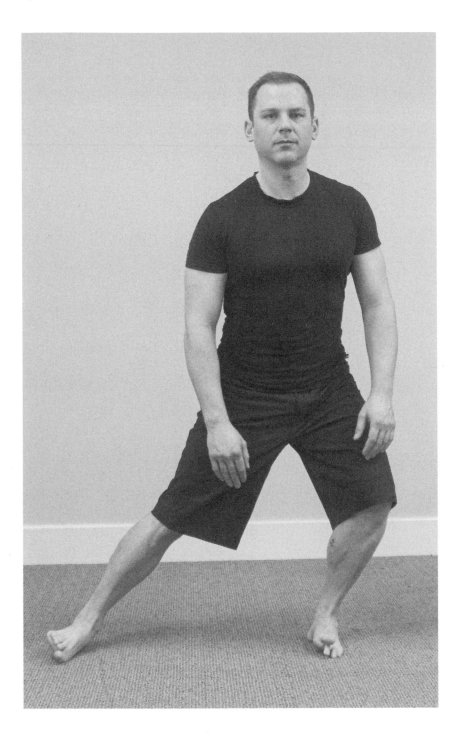

step 3. Sway the body in the opposite direction, rising up onto the other side of your feet. Repeat this slowly five times in each direction. ❀

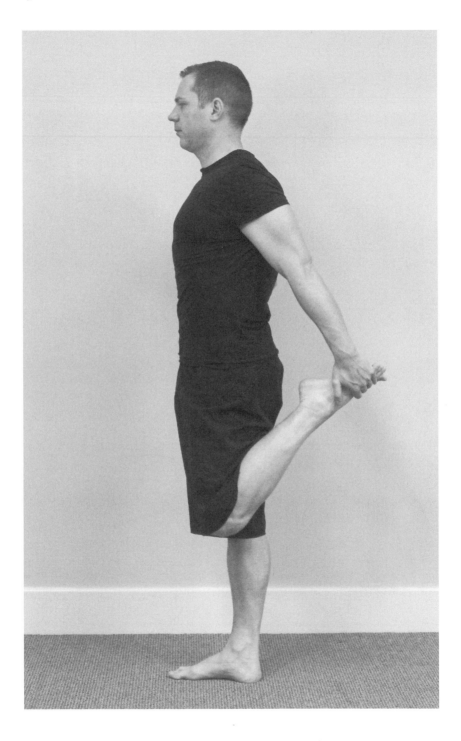

Exercise 2 / Versions A and B

There are two ways to perform this exercise.

Version A

step 1. Hold one foot up with one hand, or rest one leg on the seat of a chair, while supporting yourself against a wall with the other hand.

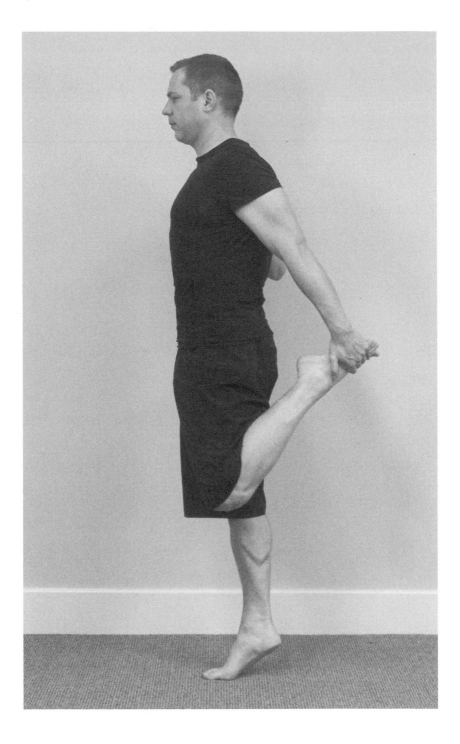

step 2. With the standing foot, come up and down on your toes, raising your heel as high as possible, then lowering your foot to the floor.

Repeat, coming up on your toes and back down about ten to fifteen times. This may cause tightness, burning, or pain in the calf muscle. This is normal, but you should stop if it's too uncomfortable.

Come to a standing position on both legs and vigorously shake the leg you just exercised to eliminate the pain, burning, or discomfort.

Repeat this exercise with the other foot. When finished, vigorously shake the leg to relax the muscles. ❀

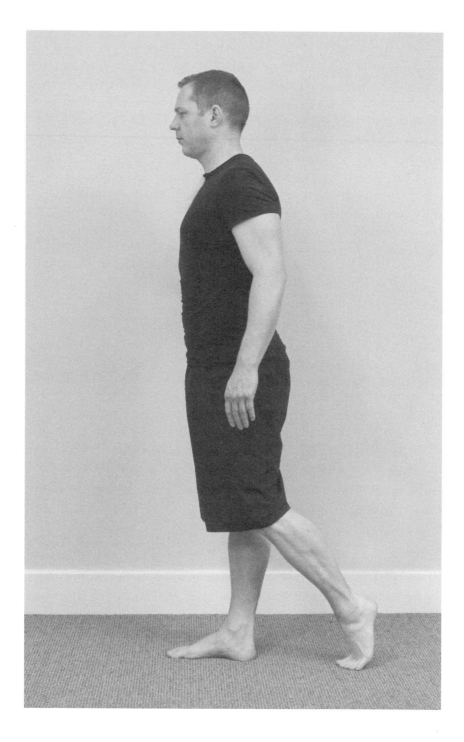

Exercise 2

Version B

step 1. Standing straight with feet together, place all your weight on one leg, relaxing the other leg slightly behind you.

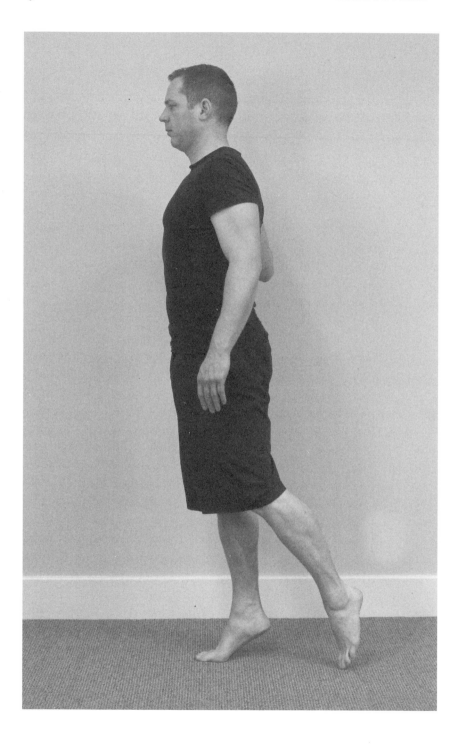

step 2. With the standing foot, come up and down on your toes, raising your heel as high as possible, then lowering your foot to the floor.

Repeat, coming up on your toes and back down about ten to fifteen times. This may cause tightness, burning, or pain in the calf muscle. This is normal, but you should stop if it's too uncomfortable.

Come to a standing position on both legs and vigorously shake the leg you just exercised to eliminate the pain, burning, or discomfort.

Repeat this exercise with the other foot. When finished, vigorously shake the leg to relax the muscles. ❀

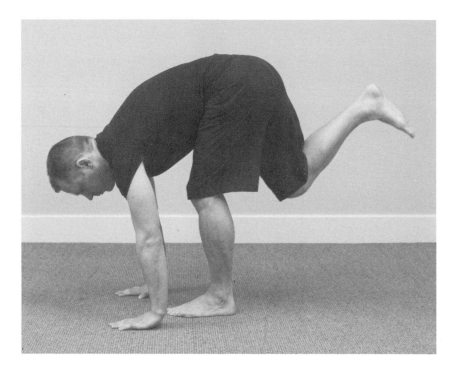

Exercise 3 / Versions A and B

There are two ways to perform this exercise. Although this is a great leg stressor and very useful, many people may find it too difficult or painful if they have problems with their knees. This exercise can be modified by holding onto the back of a chair or onto a wall rather than bending down to the floor. If this is too difficult even when using a chair or the wall, please consider the exercise optional and move onto the next one.

Version A

step 1. Slowly bend forward placing both hands on the floor.

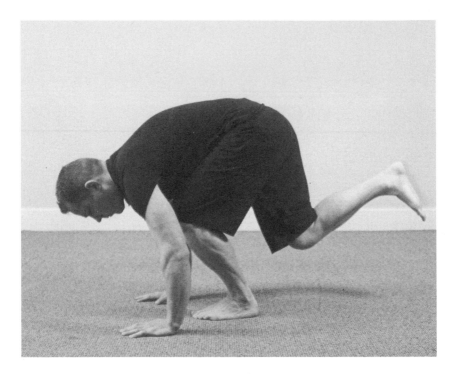

step 2. Next, bend your standing knee only as far as you can while keeping your foot flat on the floor.

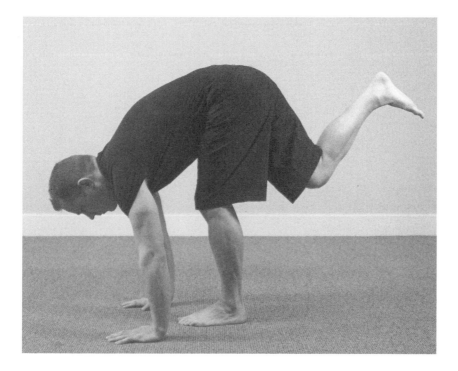

step 3. Then straighten the supporting leg. Repeat this ten to fifteen times, depending on the strength of your legs. ✿

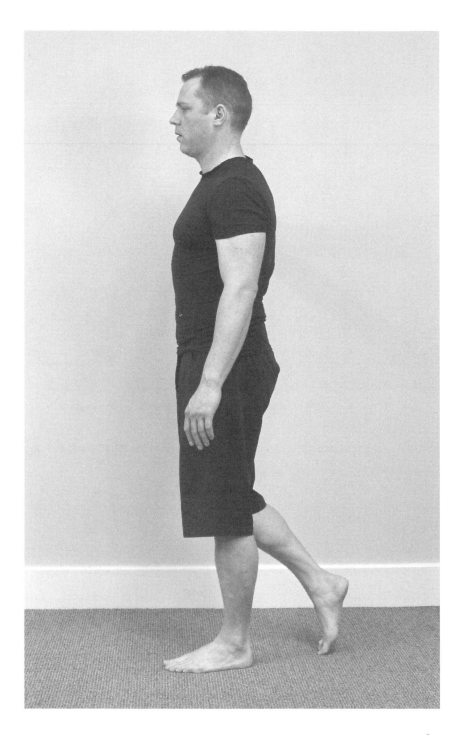

Exercise 3

Version B

step 1. While holding onto a wall or chair for balance, take your weight off one leg and relax it slightly behind you.

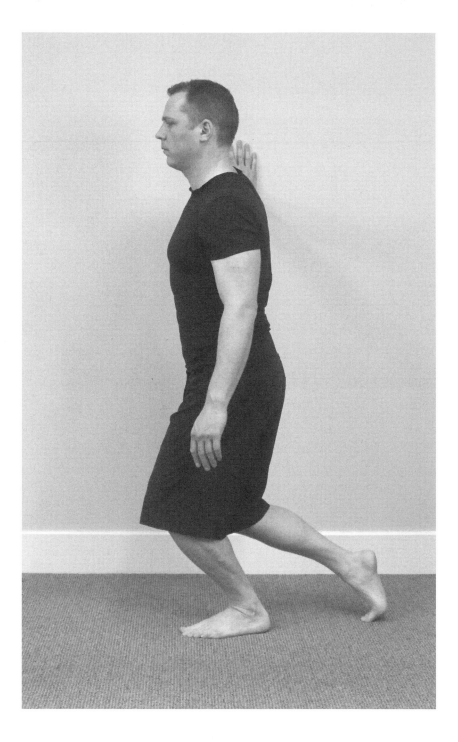

step 2. Bend your standing leg as comfortably as possible and then straighten it. Repeat this about five times. ❀

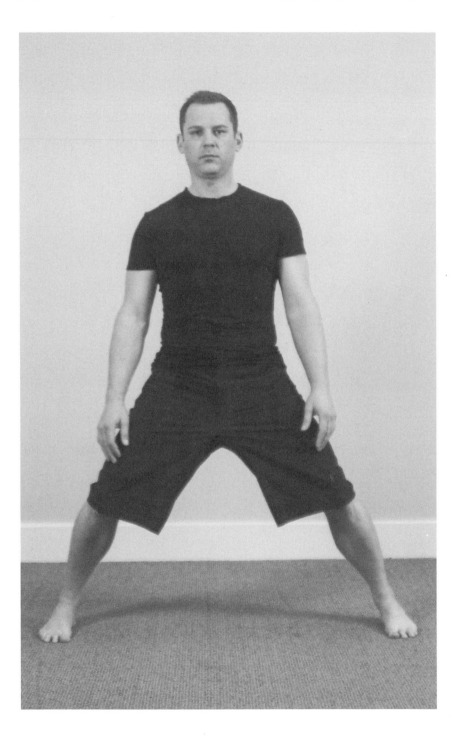

Exercise 4

step 1. Stand with your legs spread apart, so that there is a stretch on the inner leg muscles.

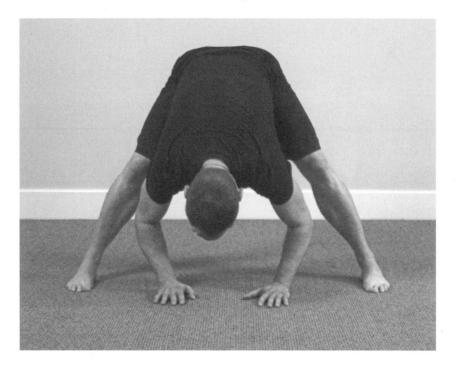

step 2. Bend forward until you touch the ground, or simply bend as far forward as is comfortably possible. You should feel a stretch on the inner thigh (adductors) and the backs of the legs (hamstrings). Hold this position for three deep breaths.

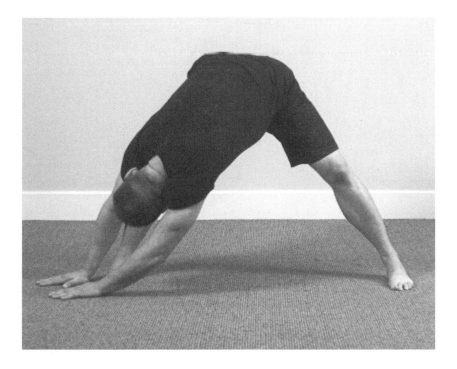

step 3. Slowly walk your hands over to one foot. Hold this position for three slow, deep breaths.

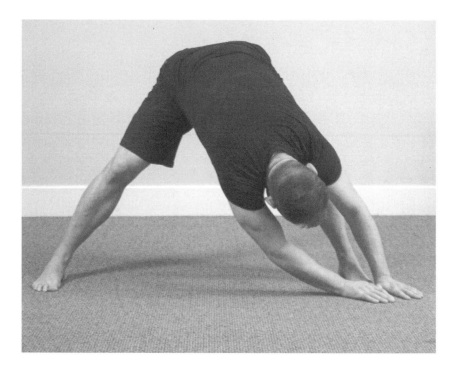

step 4. Then walk your hands over to the other foot. Again, hold this position for three deep breaths.

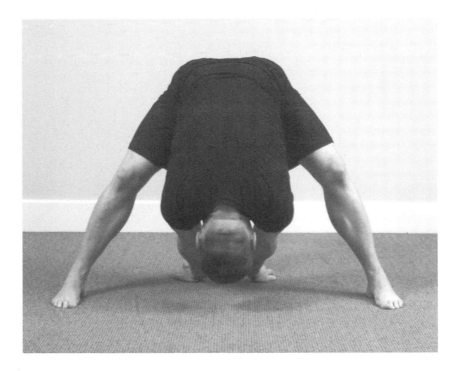

step 5. Next walk your hands back to the middle of your legs and reach behind you, between your legs. Hold this position for three deep breaths. You might begin to feel some mild shaking in your legs. Allow this to happen. To complete the exercise, slowly come back into a standing position. ❀

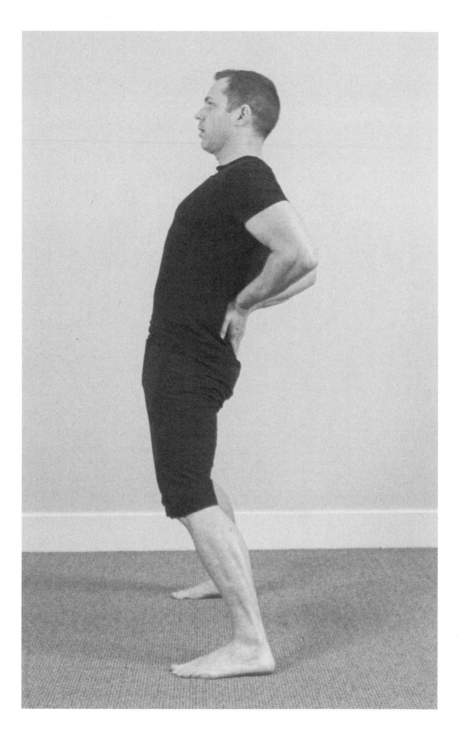

Exercise 5

step 1. Place your hands in the arch of your lower back, on the top of your buttocks, to provide support for this next exercise.

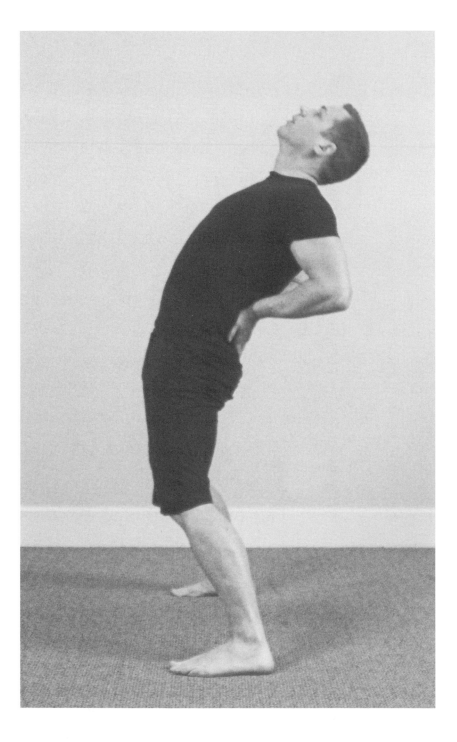

step 2. Push your pelvis slightly forward, so that there is a gentle bow in your back. You should feel a stretch at the front of your thigh. Hold this position for three slow, deep breaths. Please do not stretch too far. It is not necessary. A gentle bow is all that you need for this exercise.

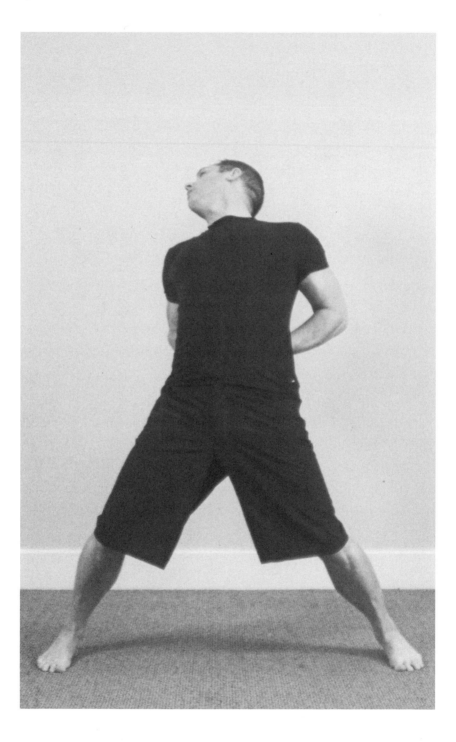

step 3. Gently twist from the hips, looking behind you in one direction. Hold this position for three slow, deep breaths.

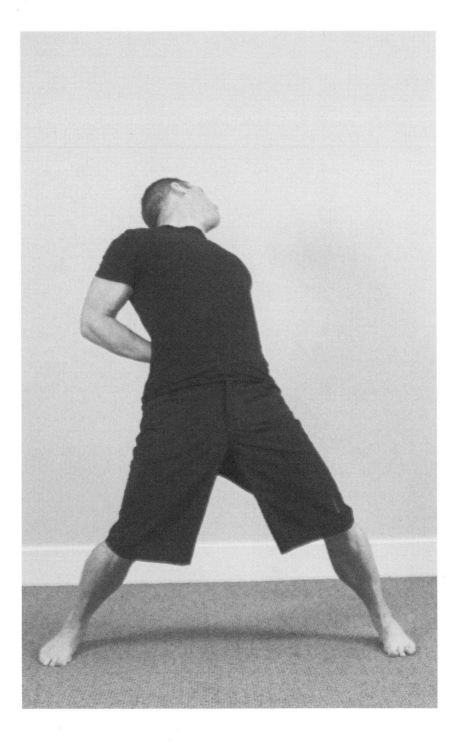

step 4. Turn again from the hips, looking behind you in the opposite direction. Hold this position for three slow, deep breaths.

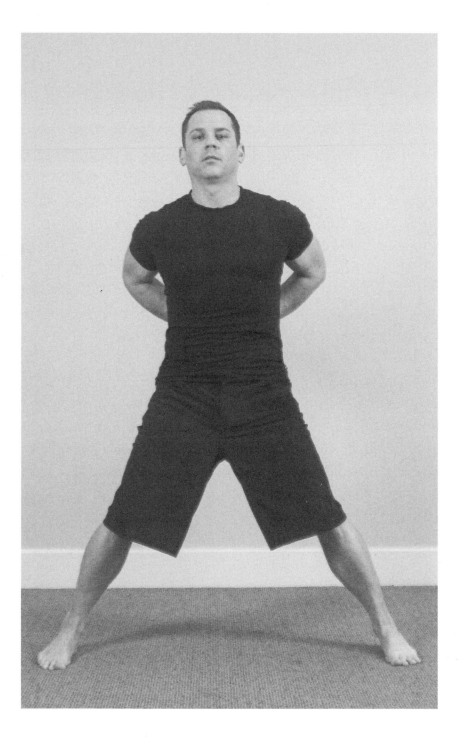

step 5. To finish, come to a standing position. Remain in a slight bow and hold this position for three slow, deep breaths. ❀

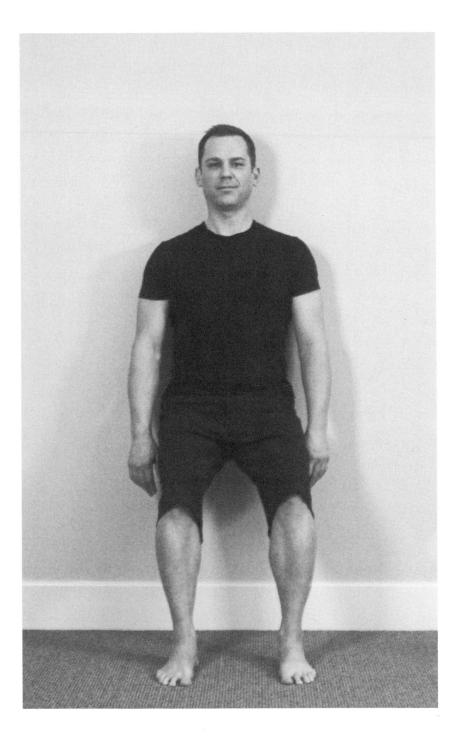

Exercise 6

step 1. Sit with your back against the wall as though you have a chair beneath you. This will put stress on the upper leg muscles (quadriceps). Only sit in a position that you feel comfortable in. Do not go too low or too high on the wall. Make sure your feet are further away from the wall than your knees. This will allow the pressure to go into the floor rather than into your knees. After a few minutes, you might begin to feel burning, tightness, or quivering in these muscles. When it becomes slightly painful, move up the wall about two more inches. The quivering may become somewhat stronger, and the pain will begin to subside. Once again, as this position becomes slightly painful, move your back up the wall two more inches. You should try to find a position where your legs are quivering and there is no pain.

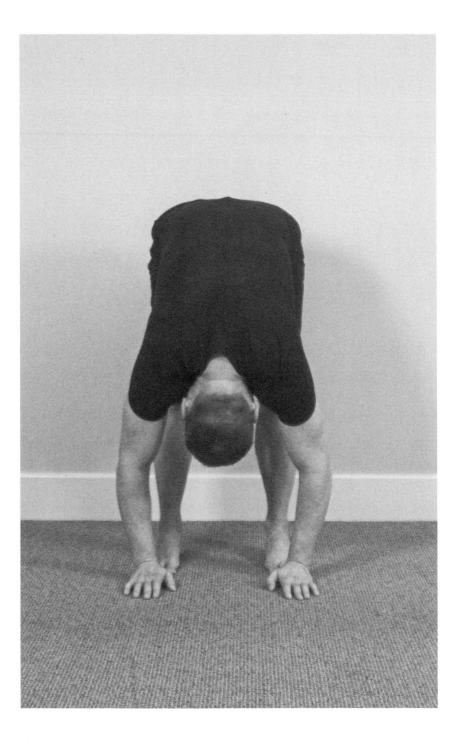

step 2. After five minutes of quivering, come off the wall and hang over forwards. Keep your knees slightly bent while you touch the ground. The quivering will most likely increase. Stay there for about two to three minutes. ❀

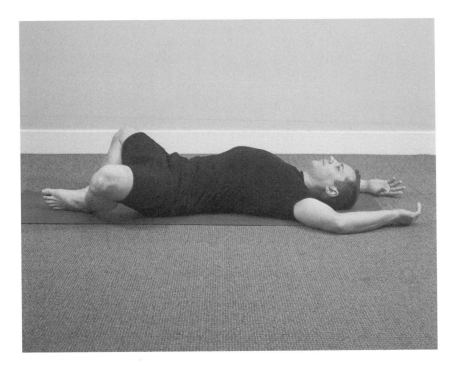

Exercise 7

step 1. Lie with your feet together and your knees relaxed in as open a position as possible.

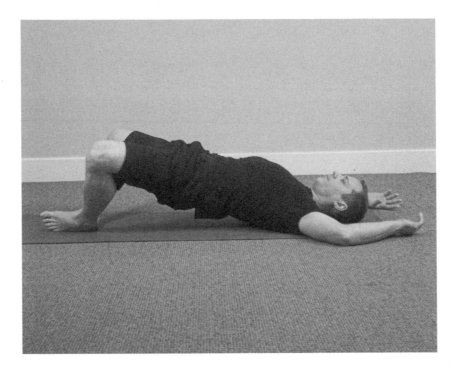

step 2. Lift your pelvis off the ground about two inches for one minute, being sure to keep your knees open and relaxed. It doesn't matter where you place your arms. They can be above your head, next to your body, or on your belly. Simply find the most comfortable position for them.

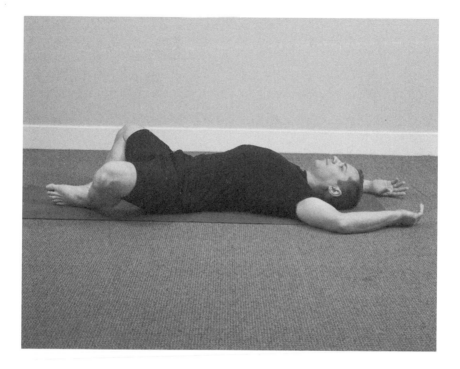

step 3. Set your pelvis down on the floor and let your knees relax open for one minute. You may begin to feel some shaking or quivering in your legs.

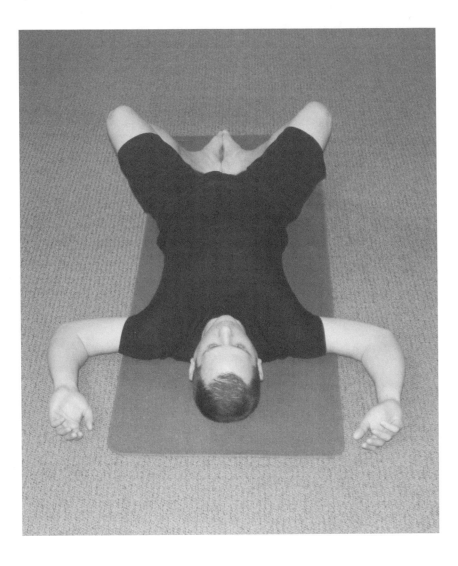

step 4. Bring your knees slightly together so they are about two inches above their relaxed open position. Lie in this position for two minutes. The quivering may become stronger. If you find it pleasant and comfortable, allow the quivering to continue. If you are uncomfortable at any time, straighten your legs and relax on the floor.

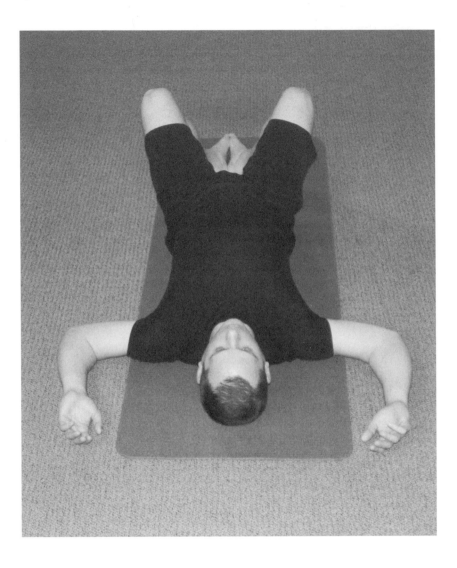

step 5. Bring your knees about two inches closer together and allow the shaking to come into your legs. The quivering will become increasingly strong. At any point, if you are uncomfortable, straighten your legs and relax on the floor.

Bring your knees about two inches closer together, and allow the shaking to continue. At this point you may allow your body to tremor for as long as you feel comfortable.

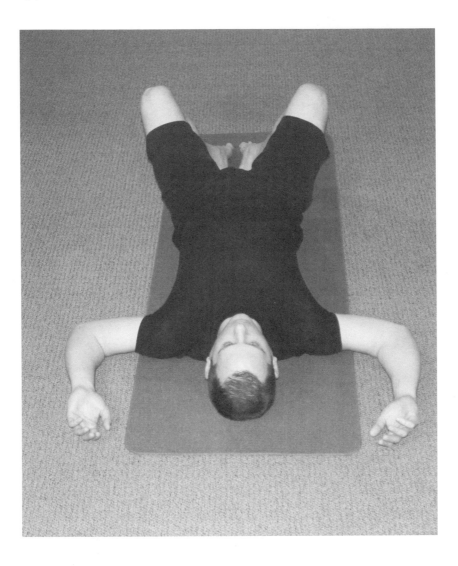

step 6. Next, turn the soles of your feet so they are flat on the floor, keeping your knees slightly apart. The shaking will continue. Allow the shaking to move into your pelvis and lower back. Remember that the longer you tremor, the more the body releases deep chronic tension. This can be fatiguing. Don't try to release all your chronic tension in one session. Moderate exercise with appropriate integration is much better for the body. If you feel your body is becoming fatigued, don't shake longer than fifteen minutes. Beyond fifteen minutes, stop at any point you experience fatigue.

To end the exercise, let your feet slide down so you are lying flat on the floor. If you prefer, you can roll over onto your side and curl up to rest. Please get up slowly and carefully, as your leg and pelvic muscles will be more relaxed after the exercises. ❀

Appendix 1
Personnel Working in Trauma Environments

THE BLACKWATER SCANDAL IN IRAQ DURING 2007, in which private American security personnel shot seventeen innocent people without provocation, highlights the importance of the appropriate supervision, training, and care for personnel in stressful situations.

It's also essential for organizations to recognize that an episode of post-traumatic stress disorder among their personnel cannot be resolved through the usual stress management programs or conflict resolution seminars. Recovery from PTSD can be an extremely complicated and intricately perplexing process. However, for a traumatologist, it's also a fairly predictable and methodical process that possesses its own logical solution.

A way for organizations to successfully circumvent the damaging effects of trauma is to provide short integrated seminars designed not only to educate personnel on trauma and its devastating effects, but also to provide them with the specific techniques necessary for prevention and recovery.

All organizations whose personnel are in trauma-inducing environments would be well advised to use the following comprehensive approach that has proven to be effective in helping to limit and resolve the traumatic symptoms of their personnel either in the assigned country or when they return home.

1. *Pre-assignment seminar.* If employees have been or are going to be exposed to traumatic situations, those employees, their senior staff, and coworkers should all be trained in trauma awareness. The individuals being assigned to regions of potential trauma should also be trained in how to use specific techniques designed to reduce the psycho-neuro-biological effects of trauma. Being able to identify trauma will assist the entire staff in coping with its adverse effects at both the personal and institutional levels.

2. *Onsite visitation.* During their assignment in a trauma environment, employees should be visited by a professional trauma consultant who can provide personal support and administer a mid-assignment assessment in a professional manner. In this way, they assess the manner in which the employees are personally being affected by trauma. They can either devise a personal plan to sustain or even improve their health during their remaining time in the trauma zone, or recommend to their senior advisor that it's necessary to temporarily or permanently remove the individual from the trauma area.

3. *Post-assignment debriefing seminar.* When the employees leave the trauma environment, they should be provided with a thorough post-assignment assessment. The trauma consultant should administer tests designed to evaluate the degree of trauma such individuals may be experiencing. This should be followed by the outlining of a thorough plan of recovery. If an effective plan is designed and

followed, employees should only require minimal reviews by the trauma consultant during the course of recovery.

This three-step prevention and recovery process is not only effective for the health of the company's personnel, it's also cost effective for the corporation. Professional awareness seminars can help to sustain employees during times of traumatic exposure, assuring their healthy and productive reintegration into the company.

Aside from the disruptive behavior of traumatized personnel, there is a growing legal consideration. A precedent has already been set by several successful lawsuits for PTSD on the grounds that the neurological changes in the brain during trauma constitute a physical injury. International corporations that have personnel living or working extensively in trauma-inducing environments are the most vulnerable to litigation. With the rapid scientific advancement in trauma studies, it is becoming more evident that trauma is the new epidemic of the international corporate world. Corporate employees who find themselves in environments that are prone to violence are going to demand that their psycho-emotional-physical health be attended to at the expense of the corporation. It will soon become standard practice for employees to file for medical benefits to cover the cost of their recovery from PTSD.

In light of this, corporations should be more proactive in protecting their employees and themselves. If dealt with in this manner rather than in a reactive manner, the traumatic experiences of employees can enhance rather than diminish their working relationships, providing a stronger and more united team and corporation. In the end, this always translates into stronger and more sensitive staff, management, and ultimately financial profitability with a humanitarian focus.

Appendix 2
The Labyrinth of Negotiation and Mediation

Sometimes post-traumatic stress is compounded by tension that has arisen between groups who are suffering from this syndrome. Similarly, tension between groups can be exacerbated if individuals within the groups are reacting to each other because of their post-traumatic stress.

This can be true of different neighborhoods, ethnicities, or groups within an organization. A large-scale example is the various parties involved in decisions about a New Orleans future in the wake of Hurricane Katrina. When tension between groups arises as it did among the various ethnicities, organizations, and political factors in New Orleans, recovery from post-traumatic stress requires a bi-communal process.

As a result of my work as a trauma therapist and third-party negotiator, I found it is safe to assume that the degree to which the participants of each group have experienced war, violence, or displacement parallels the degree of post-traumatic stress disorder that will need attention in the negotiation and mediation process.

It's important to understand that our behavior, actions, and reactions during traumatic experiences are mostly autonomic and instinctual rather than calculated and conscious. For this reason, trauma reprocessing cannot always be dealt with via the same logical and systematic methods used in conflict resolution.

I have come to recognize there are certain neurological and biological impediments in traumatized individuals that make it difficult for them to participate in the oftentimes delicate task of conflict resolution. These people should not be excluded from such processes, but should be assisted in recognizing their impediments and in gaining a greater awareness of how to deal with traumatic symptoms when they arise.

Some issues are better dealt with among members of the same group prior to introducing them into a bi-communal process. Allowing time for the individual groups to redefine themselves and practice new interpersonal and relational skills can greatly enhance the negotiation processes of bi-communal groups. Unless the groups have dealt with the issue of self-safety before they meet together, their participation in mixed groups may be premature and therefore covertly undermined by their unconscious fears and trauma-induced behavior. The conflict resolution professional will spend many frustrating hours trying to sort out the multiplicity of psycho-emotional problems that are layered beneath the group dynamics, but which ironically grew insidiously and systematically right before their eyes. If these two issues of environmental and self-safety are dealt with first, they can be used as a foundation for relationship building between the two groups.

Oftentimes the participants don't understand why they are experiencing symptoms of emotional outbursts or withdrawal. For this reason, I have often found it useful to include some trauma awareness education and simple group recovery processes to assist the negotiating parties in understanding each other's experiences. The combination of these two modalities has helped immeasurably to bring about a stronger sense of unity, understanding, and identification of shared pain. It has often been the foundation of a mutual identification of the two groups as they begin to recognize and accept the pain and suffering experienced by everyone during times of trauma.

By publicly acknowledging unresolved emotional issues, the negotiator provides a framework for understanding and supporting individuals who are experiencing a loss of emotional control. Each person's trauma may need some degree of individual consideration. For example, those whose family members have been killed in a bombing are likely to need more time to resolve their psycho-emotional pain than someone whose distant acquaintances were wounded in the violence. Meeting as a group allows the group members to assist each other in actively working with this behavior rather than viewing it as an obstacle to the group process. Meeting in groups also offers the opportunity to repair damaged levels of trust. Just as the individuals in each group must discover a new identity as trauma survivors, so must the groups as a whole redefine themselves as trauma survivors.

In her groundbreaking work on trauma recovery, Judith Herman outlines a process that establishes the need for safety as an essential element of a healthy recovery from PTSD among such groups. Instead of attempting to facilitate meetings designed to help those suffering from PTSD in unfamiliar settings such as neutral zones or third-party locations, it's more prudent for the individuals to initially meet in familiar surroundings. This is reassuring to the traumatized participants.

When the two groups are brought together, inevitably they will discover they have many experiences in common, including the fact that they are both in the process of healing deep emotional pain and memories. This can be a bonding experience for the individuals in the groups. Sharing an identity can have a powerful impact on the individuals and help dispel the image of the "other" as the "enemy." Dispelling the image of the other group as the enemy is not only essential for healing, it can be the nexus for the creation of a collective vision.

I have found that post-traumatic stress reactions and behavior can be used to build alliances across opposing sides, rather than causing them to break down into additional contentious relationships. To build such alliances should be an unremitting goal for every third-party negotiator as they begin their process of skillfully and sensitively assisting others through the labyrinth of negotiation and mediation.

Appendix 3
A Vibrational Approach

ANOTHER APPROACH THAT HAS DEVELOPED around the principle of body tremors comes from sports science. This field of study is known as *vibrational* therapy.

The first serious application of vibrational therapy on humans was by Russian scientist Vladimir Nazarov in the 1970s on gymnasts in training for the Olympics. Since then, numerous studies have demonstrated that low-amplitude and low-frequency mechanical stimulation of the neuromuscular system has positive effects on athletic performance. For many years it was primarily used by elite athletes to help increase the strength and coordination of the musculoskeletal and nervous systems, as well as to increase the rate at which athletic injuries healed.

Over time, vibrational therapy has developed as a serious field of research known as Biomechanical Stimulation. It is used in physical therapy and rehabilitation programs to correct restricted body mobility, range of motion, the coordination of musculoskeletal and nervous systems, and to accelerate the rate at which injuries heal.

This research has demonstrated that exposure to vibration frequencies between 20–50H$_z$ increases bone density in animals. It's also helpful with pain relief and in the healing of tendons and muscles. Vibrational stimulation between 50–150 H_z has been found to relieve suffering in 82% of persons with acute and chronic pain.

Animal tremors, human tremors, vibrational therapy, and bio-mechanical stimulation all suggest that vibrational stimulation may possess not only healing properties but also survival benefits.

The Trauma Release Process™ has managed to bridge the gap between animal tremors and human tremors. It has also released the individual from needing particular mechanical approaches to produce the healing effects of internal vibrational stimulation, as mentioned above. The Trauma Release Process™ is a way to reduce symptoms through the elicitation of natural body tremors. This has opened the scientific possibility for a new approach to stress and trauma reduction.

This approach does not require cultural or social awareness or sensitivity because the tremors are generic to the human species and not dependent on certain values, morals, training, or a system of beliefs in order to be effective. They can therefore be used for healing in any culture, regardless of its politics or religion.

Because the Trauma Release Process™ can be used with large populations, it is one answer to the massive trauma that is occurring on the planet. Large populations can be trained in an immediate self-help process that can reduce the aftereffects of post-traumatic stress disorder.

Endnotes

1. Bremner, J. Douglas. *The Invisible Epidemic: Post-Traumatic Stress Disorder, Memory and the Brain.* www.thedoctorwillseeyounow.com/ articles/behavior/ ptsd_4, 2002.

2. Nietzsche, Friedrich. *Untimely Meditations.* United Kingdom: Cambridge University Press, 1983.

3. Koch, Liz. *The Psoas Book.* Felton, CA: Guinea Pig Publications, 1981.

4. Levine, Peter. *Waking the tiger: Healing trauma: The innate capacity to transform overwhelming experiences.* Berkeley, CA: North Atlantic Books, 1997, 18.

5. Ibid.

6. Ibid.

7. Carbonnel, Joel. "The Umbrella Muscle." *Positive Health Magazine.* February 2000, 49.

8. Sztompka, Piotr. "Cultural trauma: the other face of social change." *European Journal of Social Theory.* 2000: 3, 449–467.

9. Herman, Judith Lewis. *Trauma and Recovery: The aftermath of violence—from domestic abuse to political terror.* New York: Basic Books, 1997, 28.

10. The discovery of this biological dimension of trauma changed public health planning to recognize the importance of defusing the chemical imbalance in the healing process. This awareness is the beginning of the bridge between

the psychological and biological aspects of trauma—or what we commonly refer to as the body-mind continuum.

11. *Diagnostic and Statistical Manual of Mental Disorders (DSM-IV-TR)*. Washington, DC: American Psychiatric Association, 2000. The manual describes post-traumatic stress disorder as situations of overwhelming stress.

12. This is called a bi-phasic or bi-modal experience.

13. Perry, Bruce D. "Childhood Trauma, the Neurobiology of Adaptation and Use-Dependent Development of the Brain: How States Become Traits." *Infant Mental Health Journal*. www.trauma-ages.com/perry96.htm.

14. See Appendix 1, 197.

15. See Appendix 2, 200.

16. Arent, Shawn M.; Landers, Daniel M.; Matt, Kathleen S.; and Etnier, Jennifer L. "Dose-response and mechanistic issues in the resistance training and affect relationship." *Journal of Sport & Exercise Psychology* 27: 92–110.

17. Holloway, Richard. *On Forgiveness*. Edinburgh, Scottland: Canongate Books, 2002, 12–13.

18. Ibid, 24.

19. Levine, Peter A. "Trauma—the Vortex of Violence." *Foundation for Human Enrichment*. www.traumahealing.com/art_trauma.html.

20. Holloway, Richard. Op. cit., 53.

21. Rothschild, Babette.; and Jarlnaes, Erik. "Nervous system imbalances and post-traumatic stress: a psycho-physical approach." Members: *European Association of Body-Psychotherapy and European Society for Traumatic Stress Studies*, 1994.